I THINK I MIGHT BE LIVING WITH ADHD, HELP!

I THINK I MIGHT BE LIVING WITH ADHD, HELP!

Nicole Skimming

Copyright © 2023 by Nicole Skimming

All rights reserved. No part of this book may be reproduced or used in any manner without written permission of the copyright owner except for the use of quotations in a book review.
For more information, contact: nicole_86@live.com

First paperback edition 2023

**Book created and published by
Nicole Skimming**

978-1-80227-995-5 (paperback)
978-1-80227-996-2 (ebook)

For my dearest sister, Danielle. I have watched you suffer living with your ADHD traits. You have been very misunderstood by others throughout your life. You are smart, and I'm sorry that people failed to see that. They failed to give you the support that you rightfully needed. I hope this book gives you relief and closure to what you have been battling with for all these years.

For my close, talented friends, Saffy Baggot, and Fanny van den Elzen. I hope this book finds you well and encourages you to find your way in tackling the few traits you have of ADHD.

Before you read on, I highly recommend listening to either classical instrumental music or white/brown noise whilst reading this book. This is because if you do have ADHD, it may stop your attention from drifting. It's worth a try, but it may not work for everyone.

Contents

Introduction 1

Part 1: Understanding A.D.H.D 7

   1. What is A.D.H.D? 9

   2. Understanding your mind in your day-to-day tasks. 25

   3. How the ways of thinking affect your potential 35

Part 2: Embracing and progressing with your traits of A.D.H.D 45

   4. Cognitive Behavioural Therapy (CBT). 47

   5. Ways to form good daily habits 67

   6. The same direction with Medication 81

Part 3: Moving forward 91

   7. Taking control of your own life 93

   8. Being open about your traits 109

   9. Life is a journey, not a destination. 127

Acknowledgements 139

References 143

Introduction

Most people say that living with Attention Deficit Hyperactivity disorder (ADHD) is challenging, especially when it comes to day-to-day tasks, such as getting ready in the morning, getting to work, and cleaning your desk or a room in the house. Are you in the middle of doing one task to then being distracted by another? Not completing one thing at a time can make some of us feel very deflated. However, some have found peace with their 'fast mind' by understanding how their mind works and what strategies support them even through the simplest task of making a cup of coffee.

If you find yourself or someone close to you with some traits such as being overwhelmed, motivationally challenged, impulsive, easily distracted and unorganised, then this book might just help you towards understanding yourself, or the person close to you, a bit more and help you manage daily tasks better.

This book is designed to give an insight into ADHD and allow all readers to build strategies that will personally help towards an easier way of living and

Nicole Skimming

'untangle those headphone wires in your mind', whether you have ADHD or not but happen to show traits of ADHD, but still need the right guidance and support.

I am not saying that all the suggested strategies will help. You may find one or two that will work for you. It took me many years and a lot of effort to make a few work. It is a process that unfortunately takes patience which is my biggest weakness, and I am still learning and working on it today! My impulsiveness trait makes this challenging. The main focus here is trying to make successful strategies a part of your daily routine and to stick with this direction of self-improvement by forming them into habits.

This book is written to be associated with adults, mainly focusing on women as they are often diagnosed later in life/well into adulthood. However, I have included experiences from different genders to share everyone's unique challenges they often face with their ADHD traits. They are to empower you to take charge of your own mind and steer you in the right direction in making your life a lot easier with the help and guidance that has worked for us.

I am 26 years old and in a loving relationship of almost 6 years. We both share a lovable 1-year-old daughter and hope to complete our family soon with a family dog. However, my life is not easy, and I have had to overcome many obstacles due to how my mind works. I guess I have always known I was a little different. From an early age, I was told that I did not listen in class and that I was underachieving, but it was never considered that I may have ADHD or dyslexia. Funnily enough, it was being diagnosed with dyslexia that lead to me finding out that I have ADHD. It wasn't until I was at university that I took it upon myself to get tested for dyslexia in my final year. I was told I also had many traits of ADHD and to follow it up with my GP. Studies show that people with learning disabilities are more likely to have ADHD. It's the same both ways. Throughout this book, you will see how ADHD is closely linked with other conditions, making it very difficult to distinguish them apart.

Although I was achieving much better in college and university, I found that I was working much harder than my peers and wondered why I was struggling so much. I would put more hours of study time in and relook at seminar classes and lectures later online for it to sink in. It would also take me much longer to write an essay and I would always be trying to make it perfect. I was not understanding why I couldn't clearly write down the information I wanted to say for everyone else to understand. Why was it making sense in my head but not clearly on paper?! It wasn't until I spoke to a class member who mentioned I should check if I had a learning disability. At first, I was quite hesitant at the idea, but she was very confident in saying that it helped her with finding easier ways to learn and articulate herself. When I was finally diagnosed with both dyslexia and ADHD, I felt like a weight had been lifted off my shoulders. I finally had a better understanding of myself, allowing me to focus on what I needed to do to find an easier way of living.

I managed to find the help I needed and eventually figured out a routine that was best for me. I learnt how important it was to set out my priorities and organise them to which most needed my attention. Using CBT and my journal helped with this and has been a lifesaver. They gave me a different perspective on managing my life and I was so happy to hear how they have worked for others too. This book will emphasise how important organising yourself can be, especially if one of your traits is being 'easily distracted'. Having good organisational skills can keep you in check and in control of your life. It may take many approaches to what works for you. But don't fret, I am optimistic that you will figure out what helps you after trialling them out with little adjustments here and there to fit your needs.

It is important to note here that ADHD isn't 'curable' nor is there a quick fix. You are not ill or the *'ugly duckling'*. Your mind just works differently. I like to best describe it like the film/book *"Divergent"* – your mind just works in too many ways and not one single way which can be a messy way of living, therefore, it's about trying to find the best way to adapt to your traits and preventing this part of you from getting in the way of you succeeding in life. I say 'traits' rather than 'symptoms' as I feel this is less intimidating and more about understanding who you are. ADHD is a part of us, so it is important to understand and embrace it and learn to integrate it into our lives instead of ignoring it and trying to cope with what can feel like a burden. I am not a doctor or a professional, just someone who feels your frustration and can understand the struggles that you may be facing and need help with. I've been there and continue to struggle at times, but the strategies in this book are ones that I have come across in my journey. Some of them have helped me immeasurably, and others not so much but I know that they have worked for other people. It isn't one size fits all.

Alongside this, it is important to note that putting strategies in place might not be enough to face the days with ease. You may also have to look at how you live your life. Your work environment, diet, sleep, hormones and relationships are also contributing factors to your ADHD and can make it more difficult to put productive strategies into practice. This book will discuss these factors, giving you more of an understanding of how we function and what is asked of us to thrive.

We are all human and I think sometimes as a society we forget that. So, as you read on and feel that you can relate, I encourage you to seek an evaluation, if you haven't already, like I did to put your mind at rest and give you the help you need on your life journey. This direction may be medication if you show numerous traits, or even choosing a different way of managing your daily life. Medication is not for everyone, but it has helped many people with traits of impulsiveness, lack of concentration, and restlessness. You may even, after reading this book, come up with your own solutions. The decision is always in your hands, and it is about finding the right one that works for you.

Part 1: Understanding A.D.H.D

1.

What is A.D.H.D?

So, what is ADHD and how might it affect you? Lucy would often find herself telling a story but the best way she could describe it was like *"explaining a road map to someone with many other routes, exits, stop points that just get in the way of the finishing point."* She would be chatting away with her boyfriend on the phone about a conversation she had with her mother that day whilst getting distracted by the kettle boiling and remembering that that was the second time she had boiled it to make herself a cup of coffee but forgot to do it. So, she would start doing that but forgetting what part of the conversation she was at with her boyfriend. She then remembers that they needed to buy more milk as she hadn't got enough for her coffee so, she asked her boyfriend to get some on the way home. Lucy also remembers that they also needed bread and other little things, so they end up talking about the shopping list. She then goes into the bathroom to see what else they needed. Lucy notices that she hasn't yet put clothes in to be washed after seeing clothes overflowing from the washing basket. Lucy starts doing that whilst remembering a funny thing her mum had said today and wanted to tell her boyfriend to only realise that when she got back into the kitchen, she hadn't taken the clothes out of the washing machine from last night. Lucy is now overwhelmed and frustrated because her mind was going far too fast for her to process and analyse which task she should prioritise first.

Lucy's traits are; easily distractible and unable to concentrate on one task at a time, excessive talking, constantly on the go and unable to sit still for long periods. These traits are commonly recognised as Attention Deficit Hyperactivity Disorder (ADHD). Lucy was diagnosed with this condition at 21 years old. However, there are many more ADHD traits and symptoms found in adolescence and adulthood.

Common ADHD traits in teenagers and adults:

- **Impulsiveness:**
  Do you often do things without giving them a second thought? Do you say something in conversation when you shouldn't have (oversharing)? Do you often get yourself in a 'f*ck it' mood and buy things without understanding the consequences in the end (struggling with money later on)? Do you find

yourself regretting these big expenses? Do you catch yourself in risky (unprotected) sexual behaviours? Do you have a sudden urge to change your room around in the middle of the night?

- **Impatient:**

  Do you catch yourself interrupting others in conversations? Are you often impatient to get things started?

- **Distractable:**

  Do you often find yourself drifting away in conversation? Are you sensitive to sound and movement which may take you away from something you were currently doing? Do you also find yourself not completing tasks because you are distracted by another task?

- **Restlessness:**

  Are you often fidgeting, never fully able to relax? Are you often feeling that something needs to be completed? This can lead to;

- **Often feeling overwhelmed:**

  Do you feel you have a lot of tasks to do that just keep piling up? Is your mind going too fast for you to process what tasks need to be completed first? This can lead to;

- **Procrastinating:**
Are you motivationally challenged to start a task for fear of feeling overwhelmed or knowing that you won't complete it? Do you have a hard time meeting deadlines and paying bills on time? Do you have a gym membership that you rarely go to? Does it take you much longer to get ready in the mornings? How long do you stay in bed delaying the day ahead? Does making yourself a coffee or having a shower feel like a never-ending task?

- **Being unfocused:**
Do you often find yourself time challenged? Do you underestimate how long a task will take? Does this make you late for things? Do you lose track of time? Do you often find yourself daydreaming when you should be listening and paying attention? Is your mind too *'loud'* for you to concentrate on one task at a time?

- **Forgetfulness:**
Do you forget appointments? Do you often forget where you have left things? Where did you place your passport or birth certificate? Do you forget conversations you've had with people? Often forget to text or email back? This links to:

- **Poor organisational skills:**
  Do you have trouble managing yourself with deadlines, appointments, or finding paperwork?

- **Achieving below average:**
  Do you feel that you should be achieving a lot higher than the grades you are getting? Or are you often questioning your progress in life in general? Should you be in a more successful position than you are now? Have past teachers or parents said that you weren't putting in the effort or paying attention?

If you relate to any of these traits, then make a note of them. This is your time now to reflect and to understand which ones you struggle with so that you can improve yourselves in your daily tasks. You may only relate to a few of these, but if you do find yourself in all of them then don't worry because sometimes just by improving yourself in one trait, you may also improve another. One example is 'poor organisational skills'. Once you can work on this trait, you may find improvements in not forgetting so much. Carrying around a diary to write down all deadlines and appointments may improve your organisational skills but whilst also help with keeping on top of them.

Louise, 31

"I was always so unorganised...I woke up every morning with a weight on my shoulders of tasks that I would keep putting off doing, mainly because I was so overwhelmed with the idea of them and didn't know which one I should prioritise first... so I would just end up procrastinating and dreading each one. I was always forgetting essential things that I would end up kicking myself after. It wasn't until I became aware of my struggles and got the help that I needed that I realised what I needed to do to help myself. At age 29 I got diagnosed with ADHD. I started writing my tasks down in a journal in order of prioritisation that I saw a difference in my well-being. I was only giving myself 1 to 3 tasks a day depending on how big they were so that I wouldn't feel so overwhelmed by them. After seeing my tasks on paper they no longer seemed so scary and what I thought would take hours of my attention and time only took between 20 to 90 minutes.... that's it! There's no feeling like the weight leaving my shoulders after crossing off each task...I wasn't forgetting things as much... remembering to call my friend and sticking to it felt like I had control again... I felt like a new

woman, a productive person in control of my life. I felt happier!

Louise started keeping a journal close by to become better organised. By doing this she became more in control of her other traits of procrastination, forgetfulness and not feeling as overwhelmed. She became more focused and therefore happier demonstrating that just by approaching one trait you can also support others. Unfortunately, one main reason why Lucy and Louise obtained their late diagnosis was that many women do not 'actively' show the signs of ADHD.

Gender difference

Studies show that boys and men get diagnosed with ADHD more often and earlier than females. This is because males show different symptoms that professionals most commonly refer to than those shown in females. This has been proven in both childhood and adulthood. Being disruptive, loud and hyperactive are symptoms mostly found in boys. These are the symptoms professionals are more often looking for when diagnosing ADHD. Lack of focus, being easily distracted and often forgetting are common traits found in girls. These symptoms are seen to be subtle and often missed by doctors, teachers and parents. Women were once stereotypically seen to be the housewife that takes on all the chores in the house such as cooking, cleaning, shopping for groceries as well as taking care of the children. Once upon a time, women would rarely come forward if they were struggling in fear of them being seen as a failure, which in turn led to very few women getting the help they rightfully needed due to not being seen by a professional and receiving a diagnosis. Although girls and women with ADHD are slowly getting recognised over recent years, it is still argued that research is still needed on the matter to improve more functional outcomes that can help them reach their potential in life.

Diagnosing ADHD

Hyperactivity, impulsivity and inattention are the ADHD symptoms that professionals look for when making the diagnosis. For Lucy, her mum took her to the GP when she was younger about her excessive fidgeting but was turned away with no further action because she did not 'tick' enough of the boxes to give her the diagnosis. She had the symptoms of inattention, but she didn't come across with much hyperactivity to make her disruptive in class or at home.

Doctors will often distinguish your traits and identify how they affect your daily duties. For example, do they stop you from getting jobs, do they stop you from making/keeping relationships, or do they stop you from achieving good grades? Unfortunately for someone like Lucy, her symptoms were often overlooked as she still took on the day with no major setbacks. She was still able to work and perform well enough for her teachers and later on, employers. However, Lucy would argue that it was a struggle for her emotionally and it became a burden for her, hence becoming very unhappy. These specifications doctors look for fail to comprehend the emotional struggles of managing these traits day to day; *"I always felt on edge, like nothing was ever completed."*

Lucy was first diagnosed with depression/anxiety but later argued that the only reason she felt this way was because of how her traits were affecting her mental state. Once Lucy got the diagnosis, she was looking for she was able to receive the right help and in turn, felt more in control of her own life and found herself much happier. Lucy shares her story to inspire others to understand their own mind and remind them that they are in control and encourage them to speak up and seek help if necessary. There are many people out there that have the same or similar struggles in which they do not fully understand how to manage themselves with their daily tasks.

ADHD is a broad diagnosis

People like myself and Lucy share similar traits but we also have different traits that also associate with ADHD. As you continue and find that you only relate yourself to a few traits, please do not feel that you should turn yourself away and not seek a professional for an evaluation in fear of them turning you away. After more research, it is now shown that around two to three out of ten individuals may struggle to focus and are unorganised but may not have the traits associated with hyperactivity and impulsiveness. The point being someone with only a few traits may still have ADHD just like someone who fits in all traits of the diagnosis. You know yourself better than anyone. Everyone is different and so, even two people who share the same traits may demonstrate their personal behaviours in their own way. For Louise, being unorganised was her main obstacle and explained how she behaved as a result. However, for others that share the trait, it might not stand out as much for them. Everyone should reflect on their own obstacles so that they can analyse them individually and see what traits and symptoms are more dominant to them and gets in the way daily. You might even already have a diagnosis but are still unsure what the next steps are. By reading this book you are already making start in taking a proactive approach to tackling your struggles.

What causes ADHD?

ADHD typically is how the brain is structured and functions. Many studies have acknowledged the differences in how the brain works with ADHD traits, however, it is not always very clear. Studies involving brain scans of those with ADHD may show having smaller areas of the brain and other areas may be larger. Other studies have argued that it all comes down to a chemical imbalance in the brain. This means the neural circuits that process our functioning of analysing information and our function to structure our memory is not properly coordinated as they would be with those who don't have ADHD. It's very untidy up there basically. Due to this imbalance, it is more difficult to problem solve when faced with tasks as our brain cannot easily access the wanted circuit. This makes it very difficult to keep attentive when it's so challenging trying to stay focused.

As well as this, a part of the brain seems to be

lacking stimulation and excitement. This means people with ADHD are likely to feel boredom more easily, therefore, they crave novelty and stimulation to try to fill in that void. Daydreaming and fidgeting are easy distractions that most people will go to when their brain isn't getting enough of it. Their mind seeks the next 'shiny' thing they see to fill in that space. This could be getting a new hobby, going to alcohol, having sex, talking, or watching tv. Literally, anything to feel stimulated.

In primary school, I would daydream constantly. I found myself drifting away in my own little world because I found it more stimulating than listening to my teacher talk. This was such a shame for me, as I have always been someone who likes to learn and has always been that annoying child of asking '*why*?' continuously. Perhaps if I just had someone take the time to communicate with me and figure out what support I needed I may have connected myself with others in the class a bit more. Instead, a few teachers believed that something was going on at home! They eventually left me to it, which is a shame, but I have a more understanding now.

It is also evident that ADHD, and its traits of it, commonly run in your genetics, usually inheriting them from your parents. Research has shown that once a child or a teen gets diagnosed with the condition, it also shines a light on the traits of the mother or father. They become aware of the traits as well which allows them to receive their diagnosis too.

Daniel, 19

"I got diagnosed with ADHD when I was 11 and a few years later I was diagnosed with dyslexia at 15 during my GCSEs. My parents took me to my GP practice and explained all the issues that they were dealing with daily. I remember ticking a questionnaire and was then referred for a specialist assessment. I remember this taking a while before I eventually received my diagnosis. I remember both my parents sat me down later that night and said they loved me, and it wasn't my fault and that they were sorry that they weren't always very patient with me… that's when they told me it was something that I had potentially inherited from my dad as he said he used to share the same behaviours."

"It did make me feel better, but I also thought I was ill and that there was something wrong with me. But I can't complain too much as my school were able to place me in smaller groups so that a teacher was able to keep me concentrated on

the tasks we were doing at the time.

I will admit that I am really bad at taking my medication now. I know I need to do better. My girlfriend often reminds me to take them, as I often misplace them. I don't know where I'd be without her, medication-less...that's where. I've lost count of the number of times I can't find something when it's right in front of me. I've become in tune with her sighing, so I know what I've done based on her cadence."

ADHD linked closely with other conditions

Studies now show that ADHD can commonly link with other conditions such as anxiety disorders, depression (like Lucy's experience), autistic spectrum disorder (ASD), bipolar disorder, Obsessive Compulsive Disorder (OCD) and dyslexia. Many anxiety symptoms exist in ADHD; constant worry, fear, panic, and sleeplessness. However, studies have shown that treating traits of ADHD may prevent anxiety and depressive disorders, and Lucy is a perfect example of this.

Unfortunately, not all health professionals can identify the difference between mental disorders and ADHD. This is because they often overlap with each other which can make them very difficult to recognise. People with depression often feel sadness, isolation, loss of interest in things they once enjoyed, low energy, unsociable, insomnia, poor appetite, weight gain/loss, and lack of concentration. Most of these symptoms can also be identified with ADHD, hence, making a diagnosis difficult. The same goes for those with bipolar disorder. They experience up and down moods, 'down' being depressive with low energy and feeling unsociable and 'up' being energetic with a higher sex drive, excessive talking and impatience. Symptoms also include irritability, paranoia, delusions, racing thoughts, unable to concentrate and poor judgement. All these often correlate with ADHD. Many people with OCD may constantly check their work over and over again trying to make it perfectly such as, re-reading an email over and over again before sending it off to telling themselves step by step how they're going to address a task. These obsessive thoughts and habits can also be associated with ADHD.

These conditions are just a few out of many. That is why we need to become aware of ourselves as much as we can in all forms; mentally, emotionally, logically and the reasoning of our day-to-day activities before we move forward with seeking help. All these conditions are a possible diagnosis for you, or it could all come down to having ADHD, or traits of it, which Lucy's case was ADHD alone. However, it is still equally possible to have ADHD alongside the conditions I have mentioned. They tend to go hand in hand. Once you become more aware of yourself, you will be able to work together with a professional on the next steps.

When I found out that I had dyslexia, it came to my attention while getting tested that I also shared the description of ADHD. Studies show that people with learning disabilities are more likely to have ADHD. It's the same both ways. Treating ADHD may assist the learning and understanding struggles of those with learning disabilities. It is always an option to treat and focus on one condition to help aid another. It is like cleaning a bedroom in your mind. You can't see or vacuum the floor without clearing out the mess in front of you first. Focus on the messiest disorder that prevents you from performing your day-to-day tasks efficiently first to allow a clearer explanation of any other concerns, or symptoms that you may also experience. This not only makes it clearer for yourself but for health professionals too for understanding the right steps moving forward.

2.

Understanding your mind in your day-to-day tasks.

To self-improve, it is essential to understand how your mind works and what particular traits set you back. By knowing your weaknesses, you are then able to work on them and form proactive strategies. Louise is a good example of this, she understood what traits needed her attention for self-improvement and acted upon them. She became more focused and happier by understanding one trait. She was then able to support the others she struggled with. Like I said, focus on the messiest trait/disorder that challenges you the most and give yourself the time to figure out what help you need.

Holly, 28

"I have struggled with anxiety for as long as I can remember. I avoided social interactions at all costs because I didn't feel like I fit in with my peers. I was constantly worrying about everything and felt so out of place. I hated school

so much and I didn't feel fully comfortable with any job I had. I did have medication eventually (beta blockers) to suppress my palpitations and it did help me relax a bit, but I then realised I was dealing with something more than just anxiety.

Once my medication slowed my mind down enough for me to think, I became easily aware of how easily distracted I was. I would be replying to emails and writing notes in meetings and still not feeling at ease so I would trail off in thought of things I hadn't done yet in fear of not doing my job right. It became evident that this constant worrying wasn't normal, and the anxiety medication wasn't the only thing going to help.

I finally went to see another doctor with the amazing support from my girlfriend and she was able to help with expressing my daily struggles from what they looked like from the outside perspective. We went down the route of ADHD and I was prescribed Ritalin (Methylphenidate)." (More info on medication in chapter 6).

Natalie, 33

"Shortly after my second son was born, I was

given anti-depressants because I was struggling with managing my day. I was constantly trying to do everything in the house whilst also being responsible for my kids. I wasn't able to think straight. I was always forgetting things from the shop, even whilst having a list in my hand. I would also forget play dates and catching up with friends. I felt constantly overwhelmed and felt guilty at the end of the day for not giving enough attention to my kids. I had no downtime. I always felt like something needed my attention but never felt accomplished with any tasks completed. I was given anti-depressants after seeing my friends with children manage life so much better than I did. They helped with my mood, but I still wasn't focused on my day.

My mother suggested that one of her students had just got diagnosed with ADHD and thought I shared similar symptoms, so she encouraged me to approach this topic with my GP. My doctor said I could carry on taking my anti-depressants with my new medication as well. I did for a while and saw amazing changes in how relaxed I felt. I felt more in control of my day…. I stopped my anti-depressants gradually and still felt good. I felt more motivated to keep a planner with me which allowed me to take

> *more things on and didn't feel overwhelmed in doing so."*

Remember it is YOUR life and you do get a say when it comes to your health. Many people forget this and place all their trust in the experts. And why wouldn't you? Of course, they're the ones that have the professional knowledge and education, so they will ultimately know more than us and have a better understanding. But sometimes they can get it wrong. We are all human at the end of the day, but you know yourself more than anyone to be in the driver's seat when receiving the help you need. If a GP starts going down the route of a possible diagnosis but you do not fully agree, then say so! Use your voice and speak up and suggest another route to take first. You don't always have to rule it out, but you can ask to focus on another direction first. It took Lucy many years to get the right diagnosis. It didn't take Holly and Natalie as long, but it still took a few years, and that's okay. It is not a quick fix and will possibly take many routes to get the right help for you. However, the purpose of this book is to speed up that process and help you become aware of yourself a lot quicker. Understanding who you are and knowing your personal needs is the key to unlocking your potential.

Do I need an evaluation?

After reading to this point in the book and feeling that you don't fully understand your mind just yet then don't fret, if you need further help with how your mind works then I encourage you to follow the next steps. You need to take time to reflect on your past experiences and understand which of the mentioned ADHD traits have stopped you from succeeding in life or have put a strain on your happiness. Understanding this will put you in control and help you to know exactly what help you need so that when you seek an evaluation, you will be confident with your understanding. Unfortunately, it is more of a challenge to fit adults into the symptom criteria of ADHD. This is because it was usually made to meet the symptoms commonly found in children which are not exactly the same in adults. The following checklist should help make this process easier for everyone.

1. Tick which traits/symptoms you have.

2. Reflect on your past experiences where they have affected you in daily occurrences such as; holding you back from performing well at school/work, affecting your relationships with friends and family, stopping you from being a responsible adult for your children, or like Lucy's case; it has no major setbacks but emotionally drains you

and can feel like you are barely holding yourself together.

3. The next step is how long have you had these symptoms? Do they start way back in childhood and were left untreated? This will give the doctor an indication if it's ADHD, or something else. This is because ADHD cannot be diagnosed if symptoms were not present as a child. It is important to note here again that this isn't an illness nor is there a quick fix. This is just simply a part of you that just needs to be managed better for you to move forward in life easier.

4. Do you have any other conditions that may resemble ADHD symptoms such as anxiety, depression, bipolar disorder or dyslexia? I will also add here could it be hormones? Hormones can make us act out of character.

5. And finally, what are your current life challenges that could be made easier for you? Again, this will help the doctor understand what you want help with the most and will often prioritise that first. This also keeps you in control of what direction you want to go in.

Step 5 is important for you to move forward on the road to self-improvement. For you to be able to understand your weaknesses will give you the best indication of how to tackle your life challenges. Becoming more in tune with your mind will give you a better understanding of what you need to personally do to make things just that little bit easier for you.

I recommend writing all this down so that you can see for yourself the reality of your struggles. It also brings out all your cluttered thoughts on paper straightened out clearly. Then take this paper with you so that you have a guideline to follow to prevent you from feeling overwhelmed, or the anxious thought of forgetting what you were going to say when you are there faced with the doctor. The last thing we want is for you to feel stressed and not in the right headspace with explaining it all.

Mathew, 29

"I was once a retail supervisor, and I was constantly getting spoken to about my performance. In busier times I wouldn't think twice about the decisions I tended to make under pressure. We were so understaffed one day, so I let one of my employee's friends help us out. At the time I knew I shouldn't really do it but didn't think too much of it. I didn't think anything bad would come of it as I was just

thinking of fixing our problem at hand first.

Once my boss found out and sat me down to go through exactly what I had done, I realised how silly it was. It was a major risk for the business which I hadn't even considered at the time. She also hadn't gone through the health and safety procedures so if anything was to happen to her, the business would be put in a difficult situation. I was about to lose my job, but instead, they understood my intentions and suspended me for 3 weeks. I was so annoyed at myself for months! I wished I had time to realise what I was doing instead of jumping straight to a decision. I went to see my GP after talking to my friend... they suggested I take Ritalin. I didn't stay on it for very long as it increased my blood pressure. I was then put on Vyvanse (Lisdexamfetamine). This allowed me to calm down and make rational decisions even during stressful times.

After a month, I saw improvements in my work ethic. I found myself no longer rushing to get things done. I took my time with tasks and was more assertive with my staff. I was a lot calmer, and the atmosphere was more chilled and relaxed. It was so nice to hear praise from them! Eventually, I was promoted to be a manager, and this was an incredible feeling as they had noticed my hard work and were happy and confident with my performance."

Mathew had admitted that his weakness had started to set him back at work. His impulsiveness often came with major consequences and disciplinary actions were made. Once Mathew understood his weakness by reflecting on his behaviours and realising, he needed support, he was able to seek the right help he needed for him to manage his work tasks more efficiently. This was his current major life challenge that he was able to grasp once he understood it by taking the time to reflect and analyse his struggle.

The goal is to become aware of your struggles and setbacks so that you can decide exactly what will help you move forward. Is the problem; work, relationships, or commuting? Could this be down to; memory, being unorganised, impulsiveness, feeling incomplete with anything you do, and being overwhelmed by certain things? Ask yourself why this could be. Dig deeper to find the origin of your obstacles. By understanding your weaknesses, you can find ways to strengthen them by deciding how to help yourself. Do you need a better strategy?

A planner? Seek out a professional? Change up your routine? Change your job? Change your environment? Basically, examining all areas of your lifestyle to find the cause of your challenges. Once you are fully aware you can create a game plan.

3.

How the ways of thinking affect your potential

Everyone I have interviewed with A.D.H.D, or traits of it, expressed how their overthinking and negative thoughts turn into self-doubt. Do you find yourself in a constant battle with giving all your time and attention to overthinking pretty much everything, including how your ADHD traits may have made the day challenging? Do you think about a social interaction you had that morning that is now on your mind for the rest of the day or week? Do you start over-analysing every small detail; did you share too much? Did you say something that may have been upsetting and now wonder if that person still likes you? Or do you overthink a mistake you made on a task which may have only been minor, but to you, it feels like another thing weighing you down because you have made it out to be much bigger than it is. This in turn leaves you feeling hopeless and incapable.

Hannah, 29

'Social interactions were and are now sometimes an initial dread for me. I have so many bad experiences of feeling out of place because I would reflect on my conversations and wonder if my hyperactivity had been too much for my friends. I would look back and wonder how often I interrupted them. Did I let them have a chance to talk or was I hogging the conversation? I would end up feeling so negative about myself. I would drill it into my mind that I was a bad friend because I perhaps forgot to ask about them or I didn't give them the chance to talk about what was new in their life.

It still didn't help or make me feel any better when my friends would reassure me when I asked about it and apologised. They would just say I was being silly, and I didn't need to say sorry but I would then think that they were just saying that. To save myself from feeling so shit and being in a low mood for days in the future, I would often avoid social outings so that I wouldn't have to be in this constant circle of torture again.

Scott, 35

"I pretty much felt incapable or too 'stupid' to do jobs. I always started a task with so much enthusiasm and approached each task at the start so optimistically that it was always so annoying for me that I could never complete them. I used to work in carpentry, and I would often catch my mind somewhere else whilst I was doing a task. My mind would drift off wondering what I also needed to do for my boss or wondering what time it was...I was missing important steps because I wasn't paying attention. I don't even understand it myself sometimes. This left the end result incomplete, and I would get told off by my boss. I would feel awful about myself for days and just tell myself how stupid I was that I couldn't even manage the basic tasks without making mistakes.

I was also a PA in my early 20s but would forget the simplest tasks of writing down the main points of a message that needed to be passed through to my boss. My self-esteem became so low that I began feeling useless at any job I applied for... so yeah, I would say it affected my potential because I couldn't stop blaming myself for being who I was."

Being too self-critical and having low self-esteem has shown to be contributing factors in stopping you move forward successfully in life. For Scott, his mind was too scattered that it was preventing him from focusing on the task at hand. As a result, he started telling himself that he was incapable of any task given to him and automatically blamed himself for every mistake. His negative thinking became a bad habit which prevented him from feeling good about the jobs he applied for. Hannah avoided social interactions because she no longer felt capable.

Blaming your ADHD, or the traits you have of it can leave you feeling hopeless. The traits you have are indeed a part of you, but you shouldn't let them define who you are. With a little support and guidance, the next chapters will give you an insight into how best we can manage our traits, so they don't consume us making us think we are incapable. The end goal is to finish this book feeling in control of your ADHD mind.

Negative thinking circle

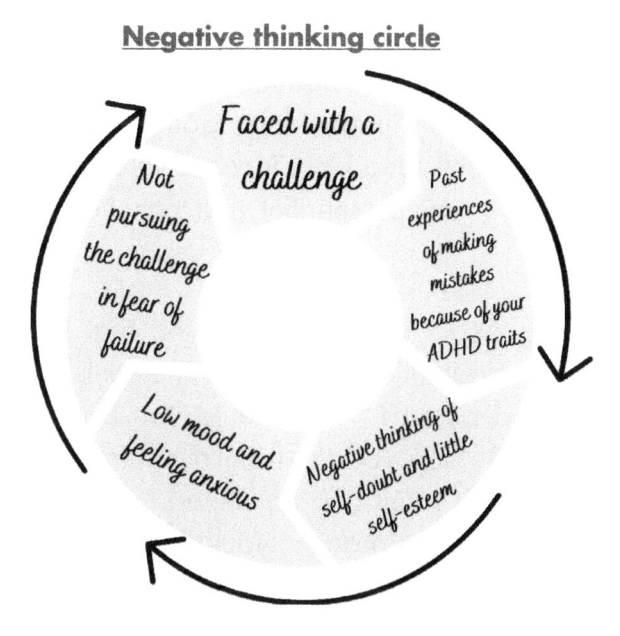

Faced with a challenge → Past experiences of making mistakes because of your ADHD traits → Negative thinking of self-doubt and little self-esteem → Low mood and feeling anxious → Not pursuing the challenge in fear of failure → (cycle repeats)

Unfortunately, as humans, we tend to focus most of our energy on negative thinking more than we do on positive. We also react strongly to outcomes that have ended badly and recall bad encounters more than praise. It is a bad habit that we continue to make. Putting all our energy into this spiral of thinking mentally drains us as a result. This stops you from positively motivating yourself to try again. To stop this, you have to redirect this bad energy and instead focus it more on a proactive positive approach. Once you become more aware of your negative thinking patterns, you can stop them at the time and change it to positive thinking by questioning your productive learning methods; how can we stop this mistake from happening again next time? How can I stop believing I am incapable? What are the strengths in my personality that can help me next time?

Thinking about applying for a job that seems out of your capabilities because of incidents that have happened before? Why should you let this get in your way?! Stop yourself from overthinking about it further at this point and go ahead and apply for it. For a positive approach, you need to realise that this is just your mind thinking negatively about it and that's all there is to it. It leaves no room for positive thoughts for you to believe you have a chance. Don't let your ADHD traits stop you from doing the things you want to do. Your mind is automatically focusing on the negative aspects rather than a 50/50 stance. This makes it very difficult to take on upcoming challenges with confidence with this kind of mindset. This will most likely lead to anxiety. You'll be too anxious to face anything out of your comfort zone.

So how do we stop this from happening? The important step is to become aware of this mindset of self-doubt and hesitation. The next is to accept and move on positively about it. What can you do to motivate yourself to apply? What will encourage you to feel good about the upcoming challenges ahead? You have every capability to take a job or task on with a positive mindset and a self-assured attitude! You don't have to ignore the self-doubt but put more of your energy on the positive side because that is what you are choosing to do. Choice plays a very important role in changing the way you think. Don't let yourself avoid a certain task or opportunity just because you have made mistakes before, that's with or without ADHD. Of course, you may make mistakes, but you will learn from them. It is so easy to let your ADHD traits consume you and define yourself as incapable, but that's your negative thinking clouding your judgement.

Imposter syndrome

Imposter syndrome happens to most of us. Often, we doubt our abilities which makes us feel like a fraud when achieving something. It is often hard for us to accept the accomplishments we've made in case of being found out. In reality, this isn't the case at all. However, we continue to argue with ourselves that we need to work harder so that we can live up to the high standards we set for ourselves. This only adds more pressure which eventually strains your emotional well-being. This can feel 10x worse when you also have ADHD. You can feel worthless and incapable. This self-doubt just pushes you towards depression, guilt and anxiety. Imposter syndrome can start from anything. It can stem from the pressures you had as a child to succeed, it can start from the mistakes you continuously seem to make, or just from seeing other people succeed. The important thing is to recognise it so that you can proactively stop this from eating you up.

Did you ever hear that saying *'fake it until you make it?* Well, it's true. Shifting your negative energy into focusing on the positive approach will start to become a healthy habit which will help you to feel much more confident in yourself and encourage you to go for things that you wouldn't have even considered before! If you truly believe that you can do something but are overwhelmed with self-doubt and being too self-critical, then tell yourself over and over again that you can do it and eventually before you know it you will already be doing it.

> "*Your beliefs become your thoughts,*
> *Your thoughts become your words,*
> *Your words become your actions,*

Your actions become habits,
Your habits become your values,
Your values become your destiny."

-Gandhi

Changing your mindset and putting proactive strategies in place will give you a better optimistic feeling, which in turn may help manage your traits. You will then have more confidence in facing the day ahead and your self-esteem boosted. This is because you will be more aware and in control. Of course, it is all easier said than done. So, how do we change negative thinking into positive processing? The first thing is becoming aware of your thought patterns. *'Fake it until you make it'* and being aware of imposter syndrome can both help for some. However, the next chapter goes into more detail about Cognitive Behavioural Therapy (CBT) which can help you change your negative thought patterns into proactive positive ones. This will also give you an insight into how to assist your ADHD traits. This is a good motivation to help you drive towards fulfilling your potential.

Part 2:
Embracing and progressing with your traits of A.D.H.D

4.

Cognitive Behavioural Therapy (CBT).

CBT is one treatment used to help with ADHD traits. Many forms of CBT have proven to be a successful non-medicated treatment that can also support the anxiety and low mood you feel from struggling with ADHD symptoms. It is a route of psychotherapy that can assist in how our minds think and react to certain events in a much better and easier way. How we process and analyse our thoughts are associated with the 'cognitive' part of CBT. Usually, thinking negatively about the tasks ahead can form bad habits like procrastination. Negative thinking can also occur when feeling overwhelmed or frustrated in certain situations; trying to plan for an important meeting, getting the kids ready and on time for school, cooking a challenging meal for your friends and family, trying to complete never-ending tasks, working on assignments for university and getting the essays completed and submitted before the deadlines can all become so overwhelming and frustrating. Annoyingly, this distress can often form anxiety which is more amplified in those with ADHD or traits of it. Resulting in negative thinking;

> *"I can't do it"*
> *"I am too stupid for this"*
> *"I am hopeless at this"*
> *"Why do I even bother"*
> *"I'm not good at anything"*

And not to be dramatic here, but I'm sure most of us have thought it; *'I'm going to jump out of the window'*. We know we're never going to actually do it but unfortunately it has become a bad coping strategy that keeps us going. We laugh but it's not funny is it really…?

How we then behave and react to our thinking is associated with the 'behavioural' part of CBT. Negative thoughts can stop you from performing your best. Not meeting deadlines for your essays, being late for work, avoiding cooking or any task again. All because we have told ourselves that we are not suited for the task. We have been conditioned to believe this way which prevents us from reaching our true potential. Continuing to behave this way results in bad habits.

Understanding your negative thoughts

So how do we change negative thinking into positive processing? CBT does not cure ADHD. Again, ADHD is not curable, but CBT can assist you with positive thinking within your day-to-day activities to help you perform better. You don't have to seek a therapist to do this. There is no reason why you can't help yourself this way. The first step is becoming aware of your thinking process. Once you become aware of thinking negatively you can start to analyse this process and work on ways to change it.

Brainstorming a thought process in a journal can help you become aware of where and when you are being too self-critical. Whether that be certain tasks, jobs, social interactions or hobbies. Write down where you are and the situation you are in; are you writing an assignment, booking a dentist appointment or applying for a job. All things that get in your way of living well. Then write down your initial thoughts on the task; this is scary, this is too difficult, I can't do this, I won't be able to do this. Then write down how this makes you feel; are you feeling anxious, overwhelmed, or stressed? Once you become aware of your negative thoughts you are then able to see what sets you back and avoid thinking this way in future.

The main focus of CBT is changing these initial thought patterns. Close your eyes and imagine you're walking through a dark and gloomy part of the woods right now. This is your negative thought process pathway. It may be cold, grey and boring. But you can stop going down this pathway if you want to. You have the power to change your way of thinking by making a new, positive pathway.

Once you find a technique stopping you from automatically going down that direction, the old pathway will slowly fade away. Eventually, you will no longer be as quick to think negatively as your new path of thinking positively will be more clear and more prominent. Your old path will eventually be overgrown with weeds and grass because you will no longer be using it! No longer visible!

You will now create your new beautiful, clean and green pathway of a better and healthier thought process. Continuously 'walking' through this new direction will become a new healthier habit. As quoted by Gandhi "actions become habits". The more you behave and act on this new optimistic thought process, the clearer and easier it will be to go to next time! Visualising a new positive pathway may help your mind go to it faster. Is the path pebbled or concrete? Is the sun shining? Is the path surrounded by greenery? Are you seeing certain flowers? For me, I follow the yellow brick road.

CBT has helped me so much. It has come in handy the most for me in varied situations;

- One, when I find myself overwhelmed with never-ending tasks such as an instruction sent from my manager, the washing piling up, needing to get petrol, preparing food for my daughter, and needing to pay bills.
- And two, when I am being too self-critical and thinking badly about myself for getting angry when I have burnt dinner because I didn't organise myself well with the timing of cooking the ingredients, or I was too distracted by things around me.

Before CBT, I would think about how much I failed that day and wouldn't be able to get myself out of that mindset affecting my mental well-being entirely. I would usually stay in bed procrastinating on what tasks needed my attention and what I should prioritise first. I would dread every task for fear of them taking too long, making a mistake, or not completing them.

It would become too much for me and I would just simply roll over in bed and sleep it off avoiding it all and hoping that it would all just go away. Obviously, my problems would still be there when I woke up, hence it eventually affecting me mentally.

<u>Using CBT</u>

Now after using many techniques of CBT, it has mostly changed my way of thinking and processing. It has slowed my mind enough for me to stop, take a breath, relax, and take a positive proactive approach to my tasks and problem-solving, instead of dwelling over them all day... even weeks on end. I have become more aware of when I am in these situations of thinking negatively about the tasks now, or how I have approached them that I am now able to use CBT techniques much sooner which has become my new routine.

Carrying a journal with me has helped me process and analyse my way of thinking to make me feel more optimistic about myself. I make three different kinds of records accordingly; a checklist for my day ahead, a brainstorm of my thinking process that needs my attention in which I find emotionally challenging, and a reflection brainstorm for tasks in which I have made mistakes.

1. A list of my daily tasks in order of prioritisation.
2. A brainstorm of my thinking process of the more complicated tasks, or obstacles I face that I personally find more stressful and bring me down emotionally.
3. A reflection brainstorm. I write down when I have made a mistake that has left me feeling inadequate, such as burning dinner or general self-doubting I would like to stop in its tracks.

The first list

I will often put in brackets next to each task if I want them completed or at least started today. I try not to overdo it with daily tasks. Just the ones that need prioritising and then everything else is just a bonus. This is so I am not overwhelmed. I then organise my day around those tasks making me feel in control and organised. For example, seeing that I have to do a food shop, wash my partner's work shirts, and prepare my daughter's lunch as my priority of the day. I will give a tick to each task as I complete them making me feel energised and in control. This way I don't feel unworthy and incapable. I won't need to think negatively about the tasks because I Know that I am taking a proactive approach to my tasks set.

Example - Checklist

Monday	Priority	Check
Food shop	(Priority)	✓✓
Wash shirts	(Priority)	✓
Take a walk		—
Prepare Lunch	(Priority)	✓
Work on my book		I did for 30 minutes - prioritise 30 minutes tomorrow
Call sister		—
Wrap present	(Priority)	✓✓
Watch film		✓

The second

Things that have happened out of your control and now have to solve such as; a pipe leak, your car breaking down, a confrontation with a friend, employee or family member, or having to make a GP or dentist appointment. The plumbing situation is a complicated task for me, so I write down the situation that we have a leak and are waiting to hear back about getting it fixed. It isn't urgent but it has been 2 days. I then ask myself is there anything I can personally do to solve the situation? Well, I am not a plumber so I cannot fix it. However, it doesn't hurt to give them a call again to ask what the update is. Once that is sorted, I then have to write it down for my own piece of my mind that the task has been solved for now and I will relook at it tomorrow to see if there are any new updates. I also write down that it doesn't help me now to stress about something that is simply out of my hands. Worrying just makes you suffer twice. This technique stops me from delaying them and I can see for myself that on paper it seems easy to do leaving me no longer feeling overwhelmed.

Example 1 – Brainstorm thinking process

We have a leak in our bathroom

Brainstorm thoughts

- What can I do to make myself feel better?
  - Call back tomorrow
  - Put down more towels

- What can I do?
  - Call them again and ask what the situation is.

- What's the worst that can happen?
  - Will we drown? No
  - Will things get damaged – potentially
  - I have to keep calling

- Is there anything else I can do?
  - No
  - I've done all that I can today

Example 2 – Brainstorm thinking process

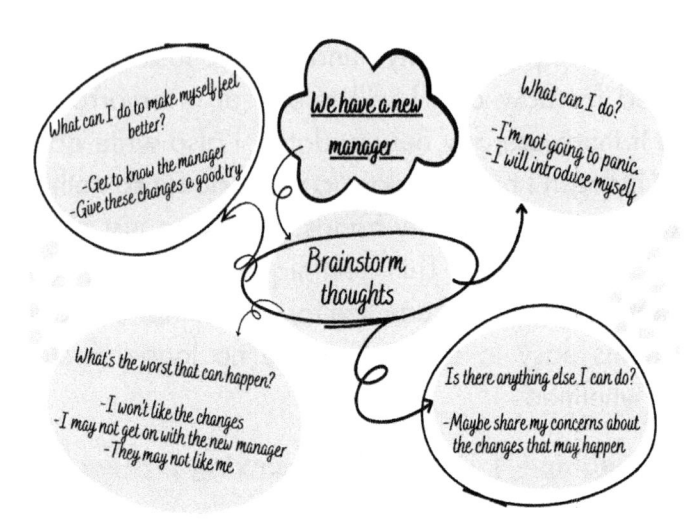

We have a new manager

Brainstorm thoughts

- What can I do to make myself feel better?
  - Get to know the manager
  - Give these changes a good try

- What can I do?
  - I'm not going to panic.
  - I will introduce myself

- What's the worst that can happen?
  - I won't like the changes
  - I may not get on with the new manager
  - They may not like me

- Is there anything else I can do?
  - Maybe share my concerns about the changes that may happen

And the third record

I write down the mistake of burning dinner and say how it made me feel. I feel angry and annoyed, even upset because I wanted it to be perfect for my family. I write down the reasons why I possibly made this mistake. The conclusions are; I lost track of the cooking times of all the ingredients I am using, such as finishing the Bolognese before I have even put the pasta on to boil. Or could the reason have been that I was easily distracted by the TV on in the background that I forget to take the garlic bread out of the oven? I reflect on all these possible reasons and analyse them so that I can better organise myself for next time. I write down that next time I would bring a little notepad with me, so I follow the cooking instructions in order with timings included. I also write that I would set timers on my phone, so I don't forget. I finally write that I will turn off the TV and anything else that could be a potential distraction. This proactive approach to reflecting and analysing changes my thinking process for the better. Instead of believing that I'm not good at cooking, I decided to take a proactive approach to learn what I could do better next time. This supports my ADHD traits and enables me to go on with my day a lot easier.

Example – Reflection brainstorm

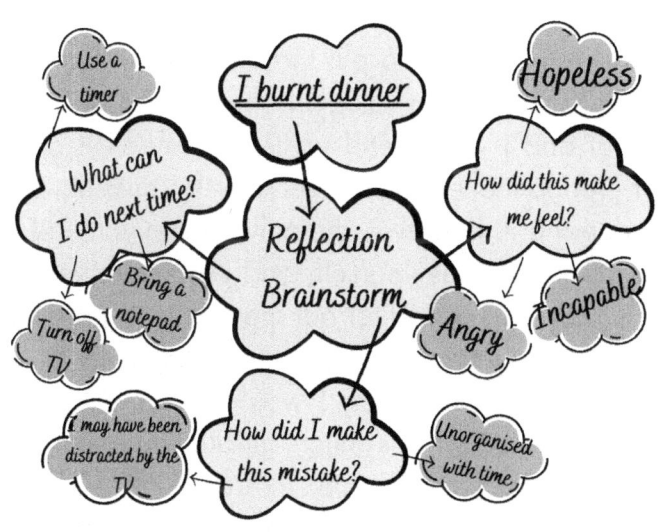

Reflection Brainstorm

- I burnt dinner
- What can I do next time?
  - Use a timer
  - Bring a notepad
  - Turn off TV
- How did this make me feel?
  - Hopeless
  - Angry
  - Incapable
- How did I make this mistake?
  - It may have been distracted by the TV
  - Unorganised with time

My journal has become my coping strategy. It helps me problem solve much easier. These lists are personal to me and are my way of implementing CBT into my day-to-day life. You may want to have your own personal lists that will suit your traits better. Writing it down on paper lets me see my problems straightened out which subsequently clears them out of my negative, untidy, and scattered mind. I no longer stress about it as I can see for myself that I took on the issue and it has been dealt with.

Using a journal or diary might not work for you, I know that others prefer to use their mind or their phone. There are also a few good apps that are useful tools to organise tasks and to use CBT. I would be lying if I said that this worked for me straight away. You do have to put the effort in and commit yourself to this new strategy. I often forgot to use my journal and I would end up telling myself it didn't work just to make myself feel better for missing days of not using it. However, the only person you end up lying to this way is yourself, and I am sure we both know that it isn't good for our mental state. I realised I was thinking negatively and not proactively doing anything about it again. I was making excuses. I became aware of this much quicker this time and brought myself back into the driver's seat and continued with it. So, eventually when you keep with it and you choose to put your time and energy into this positive thinking, this healthier lifestyle, will later down the line become a healthy habit and help you flourish into the person you aspire to be. No longer feeling incapable of doing things just because of how your mind works. You are choosing to take a proactive role in your own life. Remember you are in control of your mind, and you can conquer anything when you put the work in regardless of how cliché this sounds, it's true!

Quite recently I started doubting myself for writing this book. I started thinking negatively about what I was doing and why I was writing a book while I had other responsibilities. I then became self-aware and realised I was going down the negative pathway of self-doubt and being too self-critical again. I then got out my journal and started writing. Why can't I be a devoted mother and write a book at the same time? I started telling myself there is no reason why I couldn't do both. I organise my time well by using the first type of list in order of prioritisation. If I don't get around to writing at least a paragraph of my book today, then I will make it a higher priority on tomorrow's list. If my daughter gets poorly or is being extra needy one day then I won't fret but I will change some tasks around because I am aware of what needs my attention the most. Looking at my journal and realising that I haven't given myself some 'me time' recently then I will make that a higher priority the following day and lower the cleaning task further down the list as I know it can wait. I won't need to stress about it because I know it's there in my journal and it will get completed eventually. I won't let my impatience get the better of me because I know I can only do so much, and I am doing my best. I act on this positive thinking by putting all my effort into my journaling and note-taking. This is the strategy that works for me, and it is now my daily habit, a healthy one which makes me feel confident in myself and in control of my life.

You don't necessarily have to use journaling or brainstorming as your only techniques of CBT. There are other exercises you can do such as; CBT apps, meditation, role-playing possible scenarios in your head when faced with difficult tasks and decisions (e.g. what's the worst thing that could possibly happen or what good will come out of it), breaking down big tasks into smaller ones for motivational purposes (e.g. negatively thinking about going to work can change by breaking the thought down into individual actions. First things first, getting out of bed, then jumping into the shower, then getting dressed...), weighing more of the good than the bad at the end of the day (what are you thankful for today, and what did you do well, ultimately losing sight of the bad thoughts and feelings). I'm sure that there are plenty more out there that many therapists have created.

Amy's technique of using CBT, 27

> "My parents and teachers never really paid much attention to me as a child, and I believed that I was very misunderstood by them. My mum would always tell me that I was too annoying for my own good and a teacher, in particular, told me that I wasn't going to go far in life. In my early teens, another teacher told me that I wasn't bright enough to understand what I was reading. Growing up, I continued to believe these things about myself and didn't feel the need to push myself to aim high. Every time I struggled with my homework I would tell myself what was the point in trying anyway because I wasn't bright enough. It got to the point that even living started to feel pointless to me. Every job or task I took on felt hopeless.
>
> Fortunately, I am in a better place now, but that's mainly because I finally got myself the

therapy I needed. It was also suggested that I may have ADHD which may have made me so misunderstood as a child. I got tested and turns out I do. Even though I was making progress over the years, I realised that all my memories and negative thinking were never fully going to go away. We finally came up with a few techniques that worked for me to change my thought patterns.

My therapist pointed out that I was at my lowest first thing in the morning before I even got out of bed. I would be thinking negatively about the day ahead and my procrastination would kick in. So, it was decided that I started leaving post-it notes of self-affirmation on my ceiling, mirror, my bedside lamp and wardrobe. These were the first things I would see every morning. I wrote things like; I am good at asking for help, I am strong, I am smart, and I am funny. If I make a mistake today, then I'll get up tomorrow and try again! It was nice for me to read them each day. It gave me the confidence I needed. Eventually, I would start referring back to these self-affirmations throughout the day whenever I started thinking negatively about things or being too self-critical.

Another helpful technique we came up with was to refer to the 'QRN'. For example, when I thought badly of myself for not doing well after my driving lesson or feeling insecure about my weight, I would refer to the 3 words;

Question – I would question this negative thought. Why am thinking this way? Did anything, in particular, influence me to think this way?

Reasonable – Is it a reasonable thought? Did I try my best? Is this a way of telling myself that I need to change something to stop feeling this way again? Am I being silly for thinking a certain way? I know I'm not fat, so I know that's unreasonable.

Next time – What will I do differently next time to prevent these intrusive thoughts? Next time I'll remember that it's a silly thought to think I'm fat. Next time I'll drink herbal tea before my driving lesson to relax to avoid mistakes.

This approach made me feel more optimistic. I use QRN daily! Eventually, I started taking better care of myself, not just mentally but physically too. I started feeling more confident with doing life. After a while, I was taking more of an interest in what I was eating and what

I was surrounding myself with. I still work on myself each day, but I guess that's the point."

Amy's new way of thinking became clearer the more she used her techniques. It became routine and she was eventually able to refer back to the affirmations without even seeing them in the morning. Amy and her therapist were able to come up with the QRN technique personalised for Amy's needs which she felt confident in using. This ultimately gave Amy a better perspective on her own life.

The point is to find which technique helps you change your automatic negative thoughts into a better outlook on the matter. This changes your behaviour and approach to the tasks at hand. And don't go thinking you won't be able to find one because that's just the negative attitude we are trying to get rid of here! There will be one you will find or maybe one you are working on right now, but this won't change overnight, and it will take time to keep with it. Some may find it more beneficial to walk away from a task when feeling too overwhelmed. Going for a walk, making a cup of tea, or colouring in a colouring book can give your mind a break. You may then feel more refreshed to take the task on again with a clear mind. This method is far more practical than telling yourself you can't do the task at hand and giving up on the spot.

The new pathway needs to be walked on a few times for it to become familiar to you. This means you need to use your new way of thinking by acting on it so that over time it becomes the new norm and a habit you are happy with. So don't give up so easily. Patience is key.

5.

Ways to form good daily habits

Now it's all good having a better thinking process which ultimately makes us feel and act better. But how do we form and stick to good habits with this new way of thinking? The main focus of this chapter is to turn your bad habits into good routinely ones and how to hold on to them to keep you on your new cleaner and healthier pathway.

It can be quite fun making a 'habit tracker' in your journal by colouring in a personalised checklist rather than ticking it off.

For example; colouring in a rainbow habit tracker:

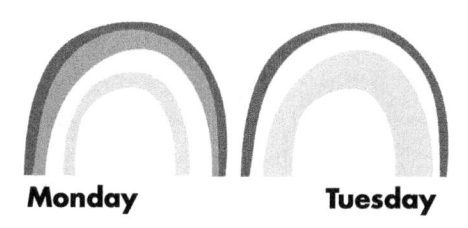

Monday   **Tuesday**

Red – Drink one litre of water

> Orange – Go for a 30-minute walk today
> Yellow – Maximum spend of £15 today
> Green – Take vitamin supplements

This technique can be motivating for some of us, however, this and the brainstorming techniques may not work for everyone. People with the impulsivity trait will find it very difficult to stick with their planning techniques which prevents them from forming good habits. Impulsive people are quicker to do things in the moment without realising the consequences at the time. Do you find yourself saying yes to staying for a few more hours at work, or agreeing to do extra shifts without realising the time you've taken away from other priorities to do this? Do you find yourself saying you'll play one more episode of your favourite series before bed, but end up watching 3 in the night, or in some cases the WHOLE series in one day leaving you with no time to be productive with the other tasks set for the day ahead? Do you continue to scroll through social media knowing you should be sleeping instead? Do you agree to one more drink with your friends when you know you should be at home getting an early night so that you are up and fresh for tomorrow's long day of work? Do you buy yourself a new bag, or order a takeaway when you know you should be budgeting?

Be your own parent

All this impulsivity of bad habits will continue to hold you back unless you put yourself back in the driver's seat. You need to be your own parent. You need to become more aware that continuing these bad habits will result in consequences for your health. Speak up for yourself and lay down the rules of when bedtime is, when to say no and what you eat.

Choice

So how do we form good habits? Over time the choices you continue to make become habits. As previously said *'Your words become your actions, your actions become habits,'* -Gandhi. Choosing to go to bed at 10 pm rather than 1/3 am over time will become a habit. Choosing to cook rather than ordering in will no longer be seen as budgeting or dieting, but as a lifestyle you've chosen to make. The choice is always in your hands.

Avoid the temptation/trigger

Delete or silence social media apps from 8 pm – 8 am to prevent the temptation. Or even turning off the notifications between this time. Organise your money into a weekly allowance and place them in envelopes to prevent overspending. By not seeing all the money together you won't be tempted to spend more than you should. You can always carry money over, but you can't use more than you have. Refusing to keep junk food in the house and deleting delivery apps on your phone will push you towards creating a new habit of cooking healthier foods and keeping in control of your money. In doing this you have removed the trigger and you will be unable to fall back into the bad habit.

<u>Delay/pause on the thought</u>

When you are offered an extra shift or to stay later at work, think about it first. Take your time to go over your journal and see if there is anything that requires more of your attention. Following this, you will be in a better position to make an informed decision about how your time will be best spent. You'll be able to avoid having to apologise to your friends and family about forgetting dinner, family game night, or the birthday drinks your friend mentioned last month. You'll also avoid disappointing yourself as this was a revision day you won't get back because it's all in your journal.

Do you ever have that feeling where you want to purchase a new phone, game, or shoes? Pause on the thought and if you can, sleep on it. Work out your finances first. Impulsive buying is the easiest way to lose money. Check other shops/websites first to see if you can get a better price. Or maybe even have something to eat. Give yourself time to let it leave your mind before you go ahead and pull the trigger on the sale as it may well be that you only wanted it right there and then. Two hours later you might not be as interested as you thought. But the following day, or even the next week, if it's something you're still sure you want to get and your finances allow it, maybe it's worth the money. Remember though, it's okay to even give yourself a week or a month to think about this decision as the expensive choice may impact you moving forwards.

I chose to delete the app 'Tiktok' because I was spending too much time on it. This helped avoid the temptation because it was no longer easily accessible.

Jessica, 27

> *"I'm a retail manager and I work non-stop. I love it! I haven't been diagnosed with ADHD, but sometimes I feel like I have it. I sometimes forget to eat lunch because I am trying to finish tasks before I run out of time that I don't...well can't stop. I can't keep still at work, I always have to*

be doing something otherwise I feel that I am slacking. But on my days off, I'm brilliant at procrastinating. I became aware that I couldn't get myself out of bed until mid-afternoon, but I was awake from 9 am. I would just be laying there thinking for an hour about what to do on my day off but never knowing what to do first. So instead, I would be scrolling through social media for the next four hours because it was easier for me to wind down after such a hectic week. I would then feel shit about myself for not doing anything productive that day.

I eventually told myself that I wasn't allowed to go on social media in the morning on my days off until I at least did one thing that was productive to stop me from feeling guilty. This could be going to the gym or a Zumba class, seeing my friends, making appointments, doing house cleaning, or doing food shopping. If I had done any of these, I wouldn't feel guilty for then jumping back into bed and going on my phone or watching 3 episodes of Stranger Things back to back."

Breaking point

It can be difficult to form and stick with good habits.

What can help, is realising your breaking point. For Jessica, staying in bed most of the day on social media was a breaking point for her as this made her feel guilty and unproductive for her other tasks. But once she became aware of this, she was able to put herself back into the driver's seat and chose to take control again. She was able to turn her bad habits into good ones by avoiding the temptation of being lost in social media and choosing to use her time more productively. This allowed her to enjoy her downtime more.

So, can you recall any breaking points that have needed your attention the most? This can be absolutely anything that has gotten in the way of your lifestyle or your happiness. Are you constantly late, unorganised, forgetful, or impulsive?

Chris (29) breaking point:

"I had my own desk, but I couldn't keep on top of anything. Staff rotas, expenses, stock invoices, health & safety and safeguarding documents are scattered everywhere. No organisation whatsoever. I became so unprepared for the business. I was at the point of losing my job until I took control of all the clutter on my desk. I bought myself draws and labels to organise

everything in its place. Once my desk was clean and I knew where everything lived, I realised I had more time on my hands. I was no longer searching all over the place for things and rushing around. I felt better in the long run. I vowed to myself that I would never let my desk get so messy again. Even now, as soon as I am aware of putting a piece of paper down on my desk, I stop at that moment and move into the cabinet. There have been times when it's gotten close again, but I always bring myself back in line. Not wanting to go back to my old ways keeps it this way. It doesn't take much of my time at all, so I just try not to procrastinate and get on with it.

This gave Chris the incentive to take control of his life and form this healthy habit so that he won't ever have to experience this setback again. This was a choice he made and is now a habit he is proud of. You won't necessarily have just one breaking point. You'll come by a few, I'm sure.

Do you remember Mathew? His breaking point was his impulsiveness previously mentioned in chapter 2. Once he realised the consequences of his mistake of almost losing his job, he made some changes and got the help he needed so he wouldn't let this trait take control again.

I remember my first ever breaking point, I was never reading or replying to emails. They kept piling up until it became too overwhelming, and I realised that they will carry on piling up until I did something about it. Not only was I living with an ADHD mind, but I was seeing a cluttered email account too. Now, as soon as I get an email, I look at it straight away and will reply there and then, or delete it if it's junk. I have been doing this for 8 years now and I can't imagine myself ever leaving an email. It's beyond me to think that I used to do that. Because I have chosen to do this for so long, it's ingrained in me that I no longer see it as a challenge. This is the whole point of forming habits. Over time, it becomes a lifestyle which doesn't need much effort.

Megan's (26) breaking point:

"Before I took medication, it was hard for me to stay focused. As a journalist, I must pay attention from the get-go. Time isn't my friend and so I always felt pushed for time. This made me skim over quite important details or stories I was going to publish mainly because I felt anxious about anything I did. Unfortunately, this made me feel that I wasn't in control, and it

showed in my work. I missed vital information at times making me look unreliable. I would also remember some information to add to the story or a question that I wanted to address to my interviewee at the most inopportune times; in the shower, drifting off to sleep, driving, or in mid-conversation with a family member or colleague. I would always just put it off at the time and tell myself there and then that I would remember to do this when I get to it, but would almost all the time forget to bring it up again. I started telling myself that my forgetful brain couldn't do anything right.

Eventually, I no longer felt in control, and it got to the point that I started feeling depressed about my job. I realised enough was enough and started taking medication. It helped me feel more relaxed and in control. I can't explain how but it did.

I also started carrying around my work journal with me everywhere and not just for the interviews. Next time a thought or question popped into my head I would take my journal out and quickly write it down before I forgot. It didn't matter that I was in the shower. Just writing my thought down in 2 minutes saved me a hell of a lot of hassle for me later. It was a challenge at the start as I would sometimes forget my journal, but I kept with it and gave myself time to sit down a few times in the day to go over it. I carried a fidget popper around with me too. This helped me stay focused and my mind busy at the same time. My ears were listening whilst keeping myself engaged. In only after a week, I felt so much happier in myself. After a month I was enjoying my job again."

Megan's inattention and forgetfulness were the breaking point she needed to take control and get the help she needed. By choosing what she needed to do, she was able to turn her bad habit into a healthier one. She was much happier as a result! As Megan pointed out, she prioritised her time in her journal a few times a day so that she would keep up with this habit. This is important for making it stick. Perhaps setting alarms on your phone twice a day so that you won't forget to do this. Or getting into the habit of looking at your journal/diary first thing in the morning and once at lunch and again before bed. This will eventually sink in, and it will become routine.

So, what are your breaking points? What habits can you make to improve your lifestyle? This is all a learning experience for yourself. If I haven't mentioned a breaking point that you're concerned about, then I ask you to sit down with a pen and paper and write down some possible healthy habits you could make to replace the bad ones from continuing. By acting now, you are taking control of your life and understanding what will make you happy. Understanding what habit will work for you is vital to succeeding in any future challenges that may come to pass. You have already started your journey by reading this far and becoming aware that your mind works differently. Even if you are just getting by now, imagine how well you would achieve if you push yourself to stick with this new lifestyle. Stop putting it off for another day, you're not getting any younger!

How to silence the bees in your mind

It can be difficult to focus on a task when your mind is craving excitement. As described earlier, those with ADHD may find it difficult to concentrate when their mind is being '*too loud*' for them to focus on what is in front of them. It can be described as having bees buzzing around in your head, annoying and inconvenient. It's not that Megan doesn't enjoy her job, it's just that her mind was craving stimulation. Megan was able to suppress this by carrying a fidget popper around with her. As a result, she was able to channel her focus by distracting the *'bees in her head'*. This means she was able to satisfy her mind whilst keeping her attention engaged.

Sensory toys

Having a fidget popper, spinner or stress ball can be used as a good mechanism for those who struggle to sit still and are inattentive. The toys fill the void of boredom allowing you to concentrate on things that demand your whole attention.

Listening to music

Loud vocal music can be quite distracting when trying to focus. However, instrumental or classical music can help relax your mind and maintain concentration and memory. Hence why I suggested listening to music whilst reading this book.

These methods can form into good habits that allow you to stay focused on the task at hand. Giving yourself the habit of journaling or writing up an essay for an hour a night with music in the background can keep you engaged and *'silence the bees'*. You don't necessarily have to just try these two. There are other forms you could try. We have all heard of white noise, but brown noise has also been shown to work for some. Find what works for you.

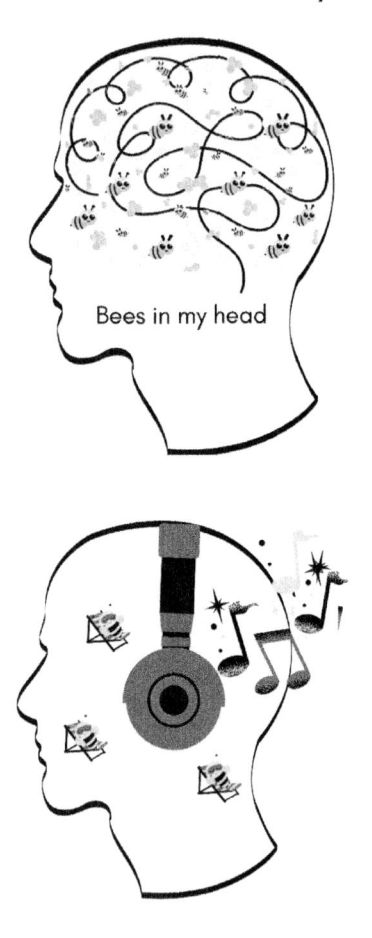

Bees in my head

6.

The same direction with Medication

Although CBT is seen to be an effective treatment approach, medication has also been proven to help with symptoms particularly found in ADHD, as well as anxiety and mood conditions. However, this isn't about taking one way or the other. You don't need to be thinking that you should just take a non-medicated route or a medicated one alone. There is nothing wrong with using both routes. You may want to try creating healthier habits as your strategy, but also want medication to help assist your concentration. Megan took the medication as well as using a journal and a fidget popper. The point is to find what works for you. Please note again here that I am not a doctor, so I don't know precisely how the medication works in the body, but from my research and understanding, I can give you an overview.

Nicole Skimming

The negative perception of medication

Unfortunately taking medication is stigmatised by society, specifically if you are taking it for your mental health. This has been an issue for many years. If you were unwell mentally, you were seen to be different from the ideal member of society. Because of this, it was common to be avoided and to have your identity changed. This affected an equal chance for employment and relationships. This discrimination could be one factor why many people were and are still reluctant to come forward to seek treatment.

Only in recent years have we started to talk about it more openly to enforce a more humane perception of it. However, why do some still suffer in silence? Is it because they see it as a weakness? Family minimising feelings? Afraid of being labelled as an attention seeker? Will there be side effects? Or does it seem as if accepting medication is also accepting failure? There are so many ways of viewing medication as a negative. However, there are also many positive outcomes to taking medication. It is important for you, and you alone to make an informed decision on what you think is best for yourself. Why should medication be seen as anything else but normal?

What is normal? We are all conformed to think and act in a certain way because society has told us to do so. But this is about understanding what is best for yourself despite what is expected of you!

Positive outcomes of taking medication

Now, of course, there have to be many positive aspects to taking medication, otherwise it wouldn't be available. There are a few different types of medications that assist with increasing concentration and staying attentive with tasks, making it easier to problem solve. These drugs are classed as stimulants. Taking this type of drug means you will rarely feel the need to seek reckless behaviour or be easily distracted by the first shiny thing you see because your brain is getting more dopamine. Dopamine is associated with pleasure, attention, motivation and excitement that the ADHD mind craves. Basically, taking these will boost what your brain chemically lacks which will in turn help make you feel more mentally fulfilled. This can help people who struggle to stay focused on one hobby without getting bored and giving it up so easily. This can also help relationships and employment.

The 3 stimulants licensed in the UK are Methylphenidate, Lisdexamfetamine, and Dexamfetamine. Although they have similarities, Lisdexamfetamine is particularly used to lessen impulsive behaviour. People who impulsively buy new equipment for a new project or hobby which they no longer stick with may benefit from this drug. Methylphenidate can also help with reducing impulsive behaviours and is most commonly used first. Lisdexamfetamine and Dexamfetamine are often the next choices if it doesn't help.

Atomoxetine is another licensed drug treated for ADHD, but it works differently than the others. This drug is classed as a non-stimulant which focuses on making the brain more chemically balanced by increasing Noradrenaline. Noradrenaline is both a hormone and a neurotransmitter. Taking this type of drug increases the chemical in the brain that it lacks. Basically put, it coordinates your neural circuits a lot easier making you function better. The goal is to make you feel more in control and organised as you will be able to access what once was an untidy mind, to locate memory and thoughts much easier and faster now that your mind is a bit more attentive.

There is the question of which is better to take. Stimulants or nonstimulants? There are pros and cons for both. Stimulants are said to work much faster than non-stimulants. They often show to work within a few hours to days, whereas non-stimulants can take weeks to be shown effective. However, everyone reacts differently to medication so what might be effective for one might not be for another.

These medications do not cure ADHD, but they can reduce the struggles you face with them daily. Taking these medications is just another way to manage your ADHD traits and help fulfil what your mind chemically lacks.

Side effects

Like every medication, there will always be a chance of side effects. They are normally the usual side effects such as headaches, dizziness, insomnia, diarrhoea, vomiting, change in appetite and more. But it is also important to note the changes in mood as another possible side effect. No one wants to have side effects. No one wants to have another thing to worry about whilst already trying to manage a problem! Of course, it would be a lot easier if it was all just a quick fix by taking a simple pill. Unfortunately, life doesn't work that way. In my experience, being aware of this sooner rather than later will keep you from giving up so quickly. It is important to take one step at a time. It can already feel like walking a tightrope when trying to get to the finishing line with the traits of ADHD. You may then see the end goal once taking the medication needed but taking it with side effects can feel like someone throwing things at you so you will lose balance again and fall off losing sight of that goal. So, if a side effect comes along while you're trying to walk a tightrope, what do we do?

Firstly, staying in control! Don't feel bullied into giving up! Get up and try again. Find a new strategy to keep you on the rope. I recommend keeping a diary when starting a new medication. This helps you stay aware of how your body reacts. Note down everything! Note what you eat, what you drink, what you do and how you feel hourly. It's important to check in on yourself regularly. Look after yourself like you would to your own child. Similar to what I have said before about being aware of your ADHD traits. This will allow you to pinpoint exactly what side effects if any, arise. You'll then be able to discuss them more with your GP. You might not necessarily need to change the drug, but perhaps change the dosage or how you take them. For example, they may suggest taking the drug with food rather than taking it on an empty stomach to prevent an upset stomach. They may suggest drinking more fluids first to prevent the headaches you've recently been experiencing as some drugs can make your body work a lot harder than normal. Again, this isn't a quick fix and may take many attempts to get it right. You are on a journey, and it is important to trust it.

Medication is your decision

After finishing this chapter and you feel that medication is the route you want to take then that's your choice. Don't let other people around you minimise your views and feelings or tell you differently. You must be confident with your own mind so that you are not easily persuaded otherwise. You are making this decision for yourself because it's your life. It's a personal choice. I'm not saying that you should ignore those that you love and trust, but it's up to you to make the final decision. You are in the driver's seat, and everyone else is in the passenger seat. If someone doesn't like it, then put them in the boot (not literally). No one knows your mind more than you do. Whatever concerns you may have with each drug, and the possible side effects that come with it can all be discussed with a professional, giving you a more confident perspective on a decision.

Megan, 26

"I now take Ritalin (Methylphenidate) three times a day. I used to take it once a day, but it wasn't enough for me after some time. I think my body started getting used to it. But oh my god does it do wonders! I felt happier and more focused in just a few days! I had a few side effects in the beginning. I had a dry mouth, and I lost my appetite, but I remember it didn't last long at all! I didn't feel anxious about leaving my house anymore or dreading the day. Even my manager asked why I seemed so much happier recently."

Holly, 28

"Taking Ritalin made my mood change entirely! Weirdly enough I also felt like they helped with my depression. I was so unsure about taking any type of drugs at first, I'm even hesitant at taking paracetamol, but I definitely vouch for this drug as I remember taking Sertraline years before and had a few side effects. I have more energy now than I ever had before."

Mathew, 29

"I went to see my GP and after weeks of assessments, they suggested I take Ritalin.

I didn't stay on it for very long as it increased my blood pressure. I was then put on Vyvanse (Lisdexamfetamine). At first, it made my heartbeat faster and I got more lightheaded, but I was functioning so much better!... After a month, I saw improvements in my work ethic. I found myself no longer rushing to get things done. I took my time with tasks and was more assertive with my staff. I was a lot calmer, and the atmosphere was more chilled and relaxed. It was so nice to hear praise from them! It was nice to be a manager they were happy and confident to work with."

Sophie, 23

"I was told that it wasn't possible to take stimulants as they would react with my other medication, so they prescribed me Strattera (Atomoxetine). My GP also said as well as taking these I should keep to a healthy diet for them to work more effectively. I don't eat much so I had to make sure I ate three meals a day so that my body kept working and digesting everything needed for my body to function. I was one of the lucky ones and didn't get any side effects. Although I wouldn't recommend taking them with alcohol. It made me have

> *unwanted thoughts and change my attitude entirely.... I didn't want to change my drugs again, so I limited my intake and had a glass of wine here and there."*

These are a few experiences that may or may not encourage you to take the medication route. No two paths are the same. No matter what route you decide to take for yourself, whether that's non-medicated, medicated, or using both as a method. You are still taking the same direction by helping yourself. Your end goal is still trying to make your life just that little bit easier. So, what does it matter what decisions you make in the end? As long as they have been chosen to suit you personally, that is all that matters. If your choice doesn't end the way you hoped, then that's okay! You just find a different method and try again. You don't necessarily have to stop medication altogether because a specific drug or dose didn't work or suited you. It may take many different doses or drugs to get you comfortable and that's okay! It's okay to feel disheartened during your journey of finding the right strategies to help you manage your symptoms/traits. Your focus is getting back on your feet and trying again until you feel comfortable. You'll get there!

Part 3:
Moving forward

7.

Taking control of your own life

Ever heard the saying that you are the main character in your own book? Well, it's true! You are the author, the main character, the narrator, the director, the leader, and the top dog! You create your own structure, your own routine. You say what will go and what will stay. You are also in control of what you eat and drink. Diet, sleep and exercise all play a part in helping ease your ADHD traits. Believe it or not, these things all contribute to helping the body function. By neglecting these necessities, you are also neglecting your health.

Making sure that you eat well, getting the right amount of sleep and keeping active, are healthy behaviours that you need to keep track of. This can be more challenging for those with ADHD, or traits of it. It can be easy to forget to make lunch when you lose track of time or lose out on sleep because your mind won't easily shut off. Making sure you eat at least three meals a day and sleep for at least eight hours a night can be seen as another weight to carry around as well as your ADHD traits. But if you don't stay in control of these necessities, it can put more strain on your ADHD traits.

As we discussed in chapter 5, it's finding how best we can form and stick to good habits, including our sleep schedule, what we eat and when. It will be more challenging to move forward in your life if you don't have control over these as well. Understanding why they are important for our body is a good start to choosing to make them stick.

<u>Sleep</u>

Although most people can get through the day with little sleep and feel okay, over time it can show effects on their mental well-being. Minimal sleep is often linked with reduced concentration, irritability, and being easily distracted. This obviously doesn't bode well with ADHD, making it more difficult to manage the traits. Over time this can disrupt your performance in tasks, conversations, and mood. Eventually, it will throw your entire routine off track. This can change how your body functions physically. You may start to find yourself more awake at night than you do during the day. This changes your appetite and mood so that you have more energy at night, making you a *'night person'* and leaving you with reduced energy during the day. Many people will then rely on energy drinks and coffee to give them that energy that their body lacks during the day. This quick fix becomes an unhealthy habit which may help at the time but defeats the major problem in the long run. The longer it carries on, the less you will feel in control of the life you lead. Your body needs a routine to stimulate all the right chemicals for the body to function.

Disrupted and irregular sleep patterns can disturb how your hormones work and the effect it has on the medication you take. Your body won't be able to regulate the production of the right chemicals effectively without having an organised rhythm. Your body won't be able to release Melatonin efficiently which is needed to encourage sleep. Leptin and Ghrelin are the other two hormones that are needed to stimulate appetite. Your body needs to sleep so that these chemical hormones can send the right signals to the brain to prepare you for food and your interest in it. Having adequate sleep also helps regulate Cortisol, which is the primary stress hormone. By not achieving this, your body will have higher levels of stress during the day. This can make your ADHD traits more unbearable to manage.

Inefficient sleep can also make it difficult for certain

medications to work effectively. If your body is more awake at night, depending on the drug, your body may be regulating it at night rather than during the day. This isn't necessarily an issue if you choose to be awake at night or you work night shifts. But for some who are to function during the day, it can be more difficult to reap the benefits when you wake up and take the medication at different times of the day. So, as well as keeping your sleep schedule, taking medication at a set time will make sure your body is regulating the drug effectively. Some people may find it easier to set alarms to take their medication and then go back to sleep, but if you are taking immediate-release medication you won't be seeing the benefits.

So how do you make sure you get the right number of hours of sleep so that you can manage your traits more efficiently? As said before, you need to be your own parent. You need to set yourself a bedtime schedule and stick to it. It is suggested that you get at least eight hours of sleep at night. However, those that can't shut off their brain as easily as others can struggle to relax.

Most babies have a nighttime routine so that their bodies and mind know it's getting close to bedtime. This routine may include, a bath, no television an hour before bed, and perhaps a story. This all helps them wind down making it easier to drift off to sleep. So why can't adults do this too? It is useful to have a regular night routine so that your body also has time to relax and wind down. Your routine may include skin care, showering, no technology before bed, reading a book, ironing your clothes for work/school for tomorrow, making your lunch for tomorrow, or having a cup of hot chocolate whilst reflecting on your day, you name it. Doing all this before bed will send signals to your brain to prepare you for sleep.

For me, I either watch a documentary like *Our Planet* or I start reading. By the end of the first page, I can barely keep my eyes open. Whereas others, they may find the book too engaging and keeping them too alert. Find whatever works for you to help structure your bedtime routine. Over time, your mind and body will come to accept this routine. Your job is to keep on top of it to make it stick. Of course, there will be odd nights here and there where you won't be able to which is completely fine. The point is to not make it become a bad habit again.

Emily, 22

> *"I've always been a night owl. I get my best thoughts and creative ideas at night! My mind*

is always racing with things to do so I often get up and draw and paint. It didn't really affect me much at first, but then I got a new job and became so tired during the day doing it. I started napping in the day after work and then sleeping in much later on my days off. Then I started getting headaches that became unbearable for me at work.

So... I tried going to bed early but my body clock was already fixed when I went to bed. I spoke with my GP, and she said that I needed to have a regular sleep pattern... so I stopped napping in the afternoon when I got home from work so that I was ready to sleep at 10 pm... I still couldn't get to sleep straight away so about half an hour before bed I would light sketch a few ideas with classical music in the background. After a few nights, I felt my body get used to it...Some nights I have to take a sleeping tablet when my mind is racing more than usual, but I don't mind because my headaches got less and less... I also noticed that I became hungry in the morning for breakfast too which I hadn't noticed before. After about a month I think, my headaches were practically gone...not sure if it was me eating better or sleeping better...I had more energy in the morning and felt I was a lot more productive at my job."

Adam, 22

"I go to bed between 1-3 am most nights and wake up sometime in the afternoon on my days off. I love sleeping in and I feel like I have more energy when I wake up… I function best when I have my full 12 hours of sleep. I eat when I first wake up, eat dinner around 6/7 pm and then I'll eat something in the early hours before I go to sleep. I remember working five 12hr shifts back-to-back once and it threw me off completely. I didn't know if I was coming or going… I was more forgetful and would become more confused than I normally am. During those days I remember not eating and I was smoking more than I knew I should. I couldn't just go straight to sleep once I finished work because my brain needed time to chill out. I was also very grouchy and moody with people and felt very restless. I never took those shifts on again."

Sleep is important and should be treated as a priority. No matter if you are more awake during the day or night, as long as you fit those hours in, your body needs time to rest and recharge itself so that you feel refreshed and alert the next day. Your body functions better if you have a set routine. This can be difficult if you work a flexible shift pattern or other obligations, but as long as you at least get enough hours of sleep to help your body function to prevent your traits from worsening.

Exercise

It is surprising to know how well exercise helps your mental and physical well-being. As most of us know, being active is good for us for many physical reasons such as; lowering the risk of bowel cancer, heart disease, and type 2 diabetes, but it also has many benefits for us mentally. Being physically active for at least 30 minutes a day, five days a week can also lower the risk of depression. When exercising, your body releases certain chemicals that can also help relieve ADHD symptoms/traits. People with ADHD lack the hormone called dopamine. As previously mentioned, dopamine is associated with pleasure, attention, motivation and excitement. Dopamine is released when participating in any form of exercise. This is another healthy unmedicated way to give what the brain needs. Sticking to a form of exercise can show improvements over time in mood, sleep, arousal, attention, motivation and memory which are all needed for our ADHD functioning. In turn, this may increase your self-esteem, making you feel happier overall.

So, exercise is needed for us mentally, but the main question that we often ask ourselves is where will we find the time to fit it into our lifestyle. A good start is finding the right type of exercise for you to ease into your day-to-day schedule without any hassle.

Finding the right type of exercise for you

You don't have to be physically fit to participate in any form of exercise. You don't always have to aim to be of an athletic skill either. The purpose could be to just take part and choose an activity that you can fit into your lifestyle. Exercise like running and cycling might not be the right type to help relieve your pressure and stress. This might suit others if they want to build their stamina, but there are other types of activities you could do to also keep active in the form of exercise. You could start with the simple, most easy ways of keeping active.

Walking

Walking is a great way to start. Walking increases energy levels and reduces stress and tension. You don't have to change much of your day-to-day schedule by fitting this type of exercise where best you can. You could choose to walk instead of getting transport to work. If this isn't possible because it is quite far and you take public transport, maybe get off a few stops before your destination and walk the rest. Use the stairs instead of taking the lift. Walk on your lunch break. Or walk for an hour after work with headphones on to stimulate dopamine into your bloodstream. Walking helps with circulation so that you reap the benefits of the hormone a lot sooner.

I used to struggle to fit the time into exercise now being a mum. I decided to look at it less as a task, but as a habit that I do with my daughter. I go to the park mostly every day anyway so that my daughter can play, but I now also make sure that I walk and push her in the pram around the whole park before or after she plays in the play area. This added 30 minutes to my day. We try to go every day so that when it's a rainy day I won't feel guilty for not going. Committing to taking my daughter helped me stick to this habit. So having someone, or a dog you can do this with can help keep this in place and make it stick.

Dancing

Zumba classes are another activity you can do with

others to make it more fun with the combination of music and dance. It can also relieve stress and tension. It can be a good laugh, but it can also be so energy-centring.

I know that when I dance, I lose myself to the music and go into my own world. This for me is the peak of my happiest. I could be dancing like a lunatic, but I don't care because I am dancing all my frustrations and worries away. It feels good and leaves me feeling energised throughout the day. Your heart rate will be faster than walking so you get to experience dopamine a lot quicker. Endorphins will be released too which is another chemical that increases pleasure, reduces stress and may also support cognitive functioning. If you don't feel comfortable dancing in public, then that's okay. I mostly dance with my daughter at home anyway and still reap the benefits. I feel a lot more focused and grounded after I have had a session with my little one. I feel more connected with others around me too and more relaxed. This is the activity for me and the exercise I highly recommend to others!

Yoga

Yoga is also a great way to help with mindfulness. It can help you become more in tune with your mind and understand how best it works under varied circumstances. Yoga can relax your mindset and help with stress relief and anxiety, improving sleep as a result. This improves your mental health as a whole, including your self-esteem. Even more, yoga can improve brain functioning, including our attention, memory, and motivation which our ADHD mind needs assistance with.

Personally, Yoga isn't my match. But that's not to say it can't be yours. I know it has helped a few people with concentration and their mood. I feel more frustrated afterwards. But like I said, one size doesn't fit all.

These are just a few healthy realistic ways of keeping active without the need to burn yourself out. Your aim is to find the right one for you that releases the right amount of dopamine for yourself so that you finish the exercise feeling good and not burnt out.

What exercise do you enjoy? What activity keeps your body moving? Once it becomes a habit, it won't be requiring much effort from yourself to do. And remember, exercise can be free, and you don't have to put yourself in financial difficulty.

Diet

Diet is another priority that we need to keep on top of. Whatever your diet may consist of it is important to have stimulated foods or supplements containing nutrients that are needed for your body to function efficiently. Different food groups stimulate different parts of the body and brain providing you with multiple forms of energy. This means, having a balanced diet is the best way to maximise your productivity.

The NHS provides an 'Eatwell Guide' for everyone to use, including one specifically made for vegans, which lays out all the foods that their body needs, including what each food group is specifically good for. Understanding what nutrients are needed for the body, such as vitamin D, iron, vitamin B12, and calcium, is important for maintaining good health.

The effects on certain foods:

Foods containing iron, such as dark green leafy vegetables, nuts and dried fruits, help with the production of red blood cells by carrying oxygen from your lungs to all parts of your body. The lack of this mineral can not only show signs of physical outcomes, but mood shifts too. Irritability and tiredness can be a result of iron deficiency. But they can also be symptoms of ADHD. Therefore, it is important to keep in control of your diet so that this doesn't put unnecessary stress on your ADHD traits. Left unmanaged, this may result in depression and anxiety. Deficiency in vitamin B12 has similar effects. As a vegan myself it can be very difficult to find foods containing a good amount of B12. Luckily, I take vitamin supplements as well as breakfast cereals, unsweetened soya drinks and nutritional yeast (which is lovely to add to almost every meal). Having this in my diet keeps me more alert and focused on my day.

I'm not going to lie, sometimes it can be hard keeping up with what exactly your body needs all the time, especially when it's that time of the month. On my period, I tend to notice that I am quicker to feel fatigued and moody, I mean, who isn't? Normally when I notice this, my body is simply asking for more foods containing iron and B12. Sometimes, my body will even crave broccoli and nuts… which I believe is my body's way of telling me what I need. When I feel like this, I will usually make more meals specialising these nutrients to keep my body functioning efficiently. When I say 'I' I mean I'll get my partner to cook. My favourites are nut roasts including loads of broccoli (roasted broccoli…I think

I may be obsessed), vegan carbonara with extra nutritional yeast and using soya cream sauce, which are enriched with the minerals my body needs. Oh, and I can't forget how much chocolate I also crave. Chocolate gives us the endorphins to make us feel good, which is definitely needed around this time.

Your body fluctuates a lot with how it functions. This is why it is so important to understand your body as best as you can so that you are aware of what exactly your body needs. Your body simply can't perform its best if your diet is lacking the minerals your body needs. How do you expect your body to have the energy and strength to make the new lifestyle changes you want when your body physically can't keep up. Energy drinks might be an easy option for getting the energy you need at the time as they're highly caffeinated, but in doing this, your body isn't getting the preferred nutrients for physical health. Hence why this is so important for keeping in control of your diet.

Unfortunately, someone who doesn't usually get hungry, or those that take certain prescribed medication that can reduce appetite, may find it difficult to ensure that they eat the right amount of nutrients. It is usually suggested to at least eat three meals a day, even if it is something little so that your body is producing the energy it needs. Keeping hydrated is also important throughout the day as a dry mouth can be another side effect of prescribed medication. People with poor time management that tend to skip meals are another factor that can make it difficult to keep in control of their diet. By knowing this as an ADHD trait of yours, you are then able to keep in control of it by creating a habit of giving yourself certain times of the day to eat. This can be done with the help of your journal and diary or set alarms on your phone. It is easy to be lost in time, so you must stick to this habit to keep in control so that you stay in good health.

8.

Being open about your traits

Although keeping a journal, taking medication, diet and exercise, and/or conforming CBT to your lifestyle may help, some ADHD traits may need more assistance. For some, making healthier habits and sticking to them may require more assistance from others as some hurdles can be harder to structure. This can make it more difficult to stay on your new healthier pathway. As said before, being impulsive and easily distracted can be very challenging to stay focused. But other surrounding factors in your life could be making your traits more of an issue irrespective of the strategies you choose. You may come to realise that you are not exactly in the right living or working environment. Your traits may be more prominent in stressful working conditions or from a dethatched home environment.

Other external factors can also be very difficult for people that have other priorities that they can't easily alter into their new lifestyle. This can be; awkward shift patterns, having children to look after, living with another health condition, or any other thing that demands their attention that we can't always control. This can make it very hard to keep healthy habits in place. Obviously, you can't just stop being a parent, or quit university, or the job you enjoy. But you can ask for help and change things around to suit your needs and there is nothing wrong with doing so. If you need an extended deadline to submit your university paper, then you shouldn't feel guilty for asking! This chapter focuses on understanding how and where best you thrive and feeling confident with sharing your traits with others so that people around you have a good understanding of how to help assist your needs with you.

Choosing your environment

By understanding your mind and body, you can adapt to the desired habitat for you. Are you in the right living situation? Are you surrounded by the right people that make you feel good about yourself? Do you feel heard and productive at work, or stressed and unorganised? Some people with ADHD may work better under pressure, whereas others may crumble and feel like they are barely making it through the day. Even using the strategies mentioned may not be enough to help. Your environment plays a huge part in your life. This is why it is so important to understand yourself and how best you function and when exactly your traits hold you back the most. You may even need to consider changing; your job, or the tasks you are given at the job, friends, time spent with family, and routine. If you don't like your current environment, then you can change your driving scenery. No one wants to be driving in an uncomfortable, clouded, and overwhelming environment. You have the power to change this. You can clear any unwanted surroundings as it's your life, your journey, and you can do whatever you want with it. You can choose any route, any direction, and any path. Once you make these necessary changes, you will then be able to focus on your new habits and new strategies without getting easily put off by the uncomfortable environment.

Job

Sometimes our job might not always match our ADHD traits. This is perfectly normal, and it shouldn't put you off what you want to do. However, this can make your job performance a little messy which can drive you crazy! If you really enjoy the job, you do but struggle to achieve your expectations, irrespective of the strategies you've tried, then the next step is to ask for help! Be open about your traits and the weaknesses alongside them. That's not to say we can't use our ADHD traits to our best advantage.

We spend most of our time at our job, so it's important for us to feel happy and comfortable there. As said in chapter 7, our job can sometimes disrupt our sleeping schedule. If you work too late or do flexible shift hours that make you work nights, it can take its toll on your traits. You might conclude that you may need to reconsider your job altogether. If you are genuinely happy with what you do, then ask for a shift alteration as Adam did. Some companies can facilitate your needs, but they may also be quite hesitant. In this case, I suggest speaking with their Occupational Health department if they have one, or a GP to discuss with them your thoughts on helping you.

In my experience, this helped me considerably. I was able to have my flexible shift pattern changed to a fixed schedule helping me sleep much better at night. Although this was done to compensate for a different condition, it still helped me perform better during the day and made my ADHD traits easier to manage, making me feel mentally happier. So, it can be done. Once you understand yourself, you can be open with them about what may help ease your struggles. You have every right to do this so please don't feel like you are being difficult. Your health and happiness come first, period! If it is an issue for them, then is this the company you want to work for?

If you are diagnosed with ADHD, then it is a personal choice to share it with your employer. Unfortunately, some companies don't fully understand it and may struggle to facilitate your needs. However, that's not to say that they aren't willing to learn. I know that there are many companies out there that will honour your concerns and will help you in the best way they can. It is amazing to see how some companies will educate themselves on circumstances like this. If you choose to hold off on sharing, perhaps you may want to share an issue with them instead.

Lucy, 27

"I worked in a bar in my early 20s and I was easily overwhelmed when it got busy and overcrowded. I couldn't concentrate on one thing at a time. I took on the job not realising this about myself, otherwise, I would have never applied. I considered leaving because it was getting too much for me. I couldn't keep focused. I really loved the people I worked with,

and our manager was always so considerate of his staff, so I was heartbroken when I told him I was looking somewhere else. When he asked why I told him how I couldn't cope well under pressure…so he suggested altering my hours from working at night to working in the day when it was less busy instead so he wouldn't have to lose me. I never even considered this to be a possibility, so I was completely over the moon when he suggested this! Of course, I said yes. I worked there for another two years and enjoyed every bit of it!

Being able to lay all your cards on the table is such a big step toward taking control of your life. Knowing what works and doesn't work well with you is one amazing step but being open about them is also a massive step that shouldn't be disregarded. Either sharing your traits, or your weaknesses is a grounded start to finding ways to work with your traits whilst having the support from your job. But as well as this, don't forget to mention your strengths! Work with them in finding ways to make you work more effectively. More examples are below;

Some traits of ADHD may be seen as a strength in certain situations:

For someone who works in an office and struggles with being easily distracted. They may find themselves distracted by the office noise of chit-chat, the machine of the printer, and the doors opening and closing. All this may prevent them from concentrating. However, if they were to suggest working from home in silence, it may boost their concentration. In turn, increasing work performance. However, this may work for one but not for another. Someone who struggles with time management may struggle to work from home. They may find that they work better under pressure, so working in the office might be the best scenario for them to make a deadline in time.

For someone who perhaps works in retail and struggles with restlessness, they may find it difficult to stay in one position for an hour or two with greeting customers or staying at the till as their attention may start to drift. But if they were given a different task of making sure the store stays clean and tidy by constantly going around it and putting things away and making it look presentable may ease this trait because they are constantly moving. Or if they were given different tasks every 30 minutes might also help with keeping attentive. By doing this, they are not only making the trait manageable, but it also becomes a strength for the person and the business.

Emily, 22

"I loved my first job at 16. I was a waitress and felt like it matched my impulsivity and restlessness traits so well. I was on my feet as soon as I started my shift until I clocked out at 11 pm. In the morning shifts, we didn't have many customers and I hated it because it was so boring and slow, and I would lose all motivation. I would start daydreaming and become very sluggish. As soon as it picked up later, I would have bursts of energy that literally couldn't be contained. I was more focused and productive. My manager would have to tell me to stop running or moving so fast because I was making him dizzy, but that's just how I liked it. I liked things snappy and felt I worked at my best this way. I was chattier and bubblier with customers. It was the perfect working environment for me. So, I asked my manager to schedule me for the evenings more than the mornings and it was no problem."

Holly, 28

"I used to work in marketing until I realised

that the job wasn't meeting my expectations. Yes, medication helped...I was on top of all my jobs and organised with my checklist once I started taking medication, but I still wasn't fully enjoying my job. I got bored easily and found myself quite restless at times. I decided to leave my job and start up my own small business... I was keeping my hands busy by making these book covers. Every time I found myself restless, I would sew and make some book covers.... Once my business kicked off, I was packaging and posting them non-stop. I was on the go from morning till night... I was a lot happier working this way."

Chris, 29

"I was extremely motivationally challenged in university. One of the reasons was that we were pretty much left to our own devices. I didn't have a clear structure for my day. I felt very disconnected in my classes. The teachers would teach, but I didn't feel engaged as a student. As a result, I was always arriving late, missing lectures, and handing my assignments in late.

It wasn't until we started doing group work that I felt more motivated. We all worked as a team to form a step-by-step structure for making a

> *project. That's when I realised, I worked better in a group. I didn't want to let people down and I had a target to work towards which kept me on track. We all encouraged each other, and I actually felt like part of a team I was proud of.*
>
> *I used the same structure of dividing tasks when it came to independent work again. I would break them down throughout my week which felt more realistic in completing them. This made it less overwhelming and felt achievable. Once I finished my degree, I started looking for jobs team driven based so that I could get the best out of me again."*

Understanding how and where best you work is the key to boosting your work performance, so don't hold back with seeking assistance and making the necessary changes. Lucy found that she didn't work so well under pressure, however, Emily did. She found that it kept her more focused. Working in the right environment for you shows how best you thrive. Being able to openly share that with your employers and colleagues can help increase your functioning. Be your own advocate and analyse the changes that need to be made.

Friends and family relationships

Relationships can feel draining whilst also managing ADHD traits. People with ADHD can find it hard to keep themselves continuously connected and grounded with others. For example, being easily distracted during conversations and constantly forgetting birthdays, events or conversations can show signs of your lack of interest in the relationship when in reality, this isn't the case. I am quite an impulsive person, so I tend to say the wrong things at the wrong time, or I will talk over someone because my mind is too fast in the conversation. This has gotten me into trouble many times in the past. I'm just so scared of forgetting what I'm waiting to say so I feel like I have to get it out as quickly as I can.

Communication

Personally, I found that being open about my traits with people and to the ones, I especially trust, helped them understand my challenges. That's not to say it would always excuse my behaviour, but it gave the relationship a foundation to work on. For example, when I would talk over my partner, he would remind me that I was talking over him again, so we figured out a course of action together to prevent this from happening. I started sitting on my hands whilst in conversation so that I was more grounded in where I was. I talk a lot with my hands too, so this gave me a second to be aware of my actions.

<u>Self-awareness of your emotions</u>

Like interrupting conversations, I always responded without self-regulating my emotions first. This is a part of my impulsiveness. I was always quick to react in the moment when I didn't like what I heard from others, or when I found the conversation too heated and stressful. Situations like these can be quite overwhelming for those with ADHD.

CBT can help you a lot in these circumstances. Changing your thought process can change your behaviour. Instead of shutting down and behaving as you always do, stop, think and analyse your negative thinking process. Then change it into something like;

> *"My manager has just said that I need to make some changes to my report, instead of initially being despondent and abrupt, I will analyse my body language and ask for what specific alterations they have in mind, and if they could break it down for me step by step so it isn't so overwhelming."*

Don't feel like you are asking for it to be 'dumbed'

down for you. There is nothing wrong with asking for support from your employer to ease your ADHD traits. A good supervisor will always want to get the best out of you. This way, you are communicating your needs and concerns. This should make it stress-free for everyone.

Another example is;

> "My sister has just said that I always forget what she tells me in our conversations. Instead of being defensive, I will sympathise with her frustration and explain my struggle at remembering things."

Remember that you are only in control of your own emotions, other people's behaviour and emotions are not your responsibility.

Seeking a resolution

Communication, and being self-aware might not always be enough in closer relationships. Sometimes coming up with a resolution like sitting on your hands whilst in conversation can be a good start but sticking to it and being committed to the changes is another step. If you say that you won't forget events or break promises, you need to actively do so. Maybe share with them the changes you'll make to prevent this from happening in the future. Will you write all events on a calendar or set a reminder set on your phone? Will you work on getting yourself seen by a professional? Will you stop impulsive spending by putting strategies in place? These are just a few examples to be considered with your family and friends to prevent tension in the relationship.

Louise, 31

"I would often forget my friend's birthdays, her children's birthdays, and her doctor appointments whilst she was pregnant. Being so unorganised made me feel like the worst friend... I would always forget to call her in the evenings when she asked. She would get so upset with me but would never really discuss it until one night when I had forgotten about her baby shower. She said she found it difficult being friends with me. It hurt a lot at the time because I just wanted her to understand that I wasn't doing it on purpose... so we didn't talk for a month. I eventually wrote her a letter in which I was able to have the time to write everything down without any distractions and I told her I went to see a doctor. She phoned a few days later and it was water under the bridge. I no longer kept her in the dark and she

began helping me... she would often remind me to add things to my journal and calendar so that I wouldn't forget... she helped me a lot through the process of getting better organised and it honestly felt like a weight had lifted from my shoulders."

Mathew, 29

"I went to see my GP after talking to my friend... he suggested that it would be best if I spoke to someone about my troubles after I told him how low I was getting. I probably wouldn't have gone if I didn't have his support or encouragement. I honestly thought I was being silly at first, but he reassured me that if it was getting me down this much then it wasn't normal, and I shouldn't suffer in silence. After a month, I saw improvements in my work ethic."

Danielle, 25

"Sometimes my boyfriend, friends and family struggle to be around me when I am having one of my hyper moments. I am excessively talking and, in their faces, because I have so much energy. Sometimes it feels like I could be bouncing off the walls. I say and do things to get a reaction from them for fun. My hyperactivity

doesn't really bother me because I know it's a part of me and it always has been, but it upsets me when the people who are close to me get annoyed or upset by my actions. My sister would often say that my behaviour was unpredictable when I was in moods like this. She always felt like she was on edge when I was being 'too much.

A few have said that they notice it more whilst I'm waiting for food, or after eating certain surgery foods. My mum would always say it after I had tomato sauce. But most of the time they can just come on at any time. My friends and family have a bit more understanding when I tell them it's my ADHD and we do laugh it off sometimes, but maybe I do need to find certain ways to calm myself down a bit."

Fatima, 34

"My ex-husband knew that I was terrible at remembering things and he was the best at using it against me. At the time, I didn't realise I was being manipulated or gaslighted. I have never been professionally diagnosed with ADHD but have always felt I have had it since childhood. I would often blame what I thought was ADHD, and never my husband for the way he treated

me and made me feel. Once I started using a planner I eventually felt on top of things. I was remembering more and felt more confident with my memory. My ex-husband would still manipulate me and make out I was stupid. That was when I realised our marriage was over."

Being open and honest with your family and friends can go a long way in helping yourself. Whether that's having a better understanding, a little encouragement, or working on resolutions to improve yourself in certain situations so that you feel more grounded with yourself and others. You don't have to work through it alone. Help should always be there when asked and you shouldn't feel guilty in doing so. If the support isn't there, then maybe you are not surrounded by the right people. It is okay to walk away from people that don't make you feel welcome or supported. ADHD is a part of you. No one in your inner circle should make you feel shitty or make you feel like the ugly duckling in any scenario. As I said, you are the main character in your own book, you can say who stays or who you decide to kill off. People who care about you would want to understand your struggles and how best to help you. But it is also important that you let them. I am not saying you have to make yourself completely vulnerable, you can if you want to, and you trust them but letting them understand you is important to carry on with the relationship you want.

9.

Life is a journey, not a destination.

From reading this far, you will hopefully by now have a rough understanding of what might help ease your ADHD traits. Life is for trying and learning what works for you. You may feel quite impatient with wanting a quick fix. It is frustrating that these changes will take time and patience. But, once you become fully aware of what particular traits and bad habits hold you back, you are then able to move forward in creating the right environment for yourself. Prioritise what you want to focus on first. You might realise that you may need to take medication to help with the habits that you want to make. It is a step-by-step process. You'll figure it out. Try and find the fun in discovering yourself, like reading a new book about who you are and the journey you're on. Life is a journey, not a destination. Enjoy the ride. There's no rush! You have the power, ability, and determination to lead the life you want. ADHD does not define you, it is simply a part of you that you are willing to explore and understand. There's no reason why your

ADHD has to hold you back!

Simone Biles is an American artistic gymnast who has had ADHD since she was a child. Yet this hasn't stopped her from succeeding and living the life she wants. She has won 32 Olympic and World Championship medals and was awarded the Presidential Medal of Freedom in 2022! She became the youngest person to receive the nation's highest civilian honour. Amazing! She feels no shame in taking medication and has been taking it since she was a child. Let her example be the confidence you need to be your own advocate!

More celebrities with ADHD:

Emma Watson
Channing Tatum
Dave Grohl
Justin Timberlake
Johnny Depp
Zooey Deschanel
Mel B

Mel B tells us that she exercises and meditates to get rid of her anxiety. Zooey has struggled with staying focused and finding it difficult to complete things that require her patience. At least four of these celebrities are also living with another condition. Don't see it as another thing being 'wrong' with you, but rather, as something else you have figured out about yourself and are willing to adjust your life to accommodate for an easier way of living. You're not alone.

Always remember that it's okay to not always be going through life in one straight line. There will be times when you will be standing still for a while to figure things out. You may then decide to take a different direction in your journey. This is normal. We are all figuring life out, but by wanting to do so in the most stress-free way possible. Once you've understood yourself, embrace it. You'll then be able to share your experience with others to help and influence them on their journey.

Rewarding yourself.

Rewarding yourself can be a way of keeping yourself in check and happy with your new lifestyle. It doesn't need to put you in financial difficulty, but rewarding yourself with something you enjoy like; reading a book with a cup of hot chocolate, playing on the Xbox or PlayStation for an hour, taking a hot bubble bath, or watching a feel-good movie. Make sure you do this often after completing a challenging task like; going to bed on time, writing in your journal, finally making that appointment, or after an exercise activity that was on your to-do-list for the day. Rewarding yourself can keep these healthy habits in place and give you the motivation to take on any challenging task.

I used to hate going for runs in the evening after work, but once I started getting into the habit of watching an episode of my favourite show afterwards, it became the normality. I stopped procrastinating about it too much and just did it. I didn't stick to it, but I did change my exercise activity to walking in the park with my daughter and that was a treat in itself as I got to spend some quality time with her. I adapted to the change and kept to the habit.

Adapting to change

Once you have a routine and the life you have worked for, it is important to note that changes along your journey can throw us off your course. Changes in your workplace, moving house, becoming a parent, and losing a loved one are all changes that we need to be prepared for.

For me, becoming a parent threw me off my routine entirely. I didn't know what day it was or when I last ate. I got into the habit of eating anything easy and something to pass me over. Luckily, I had the incentive to keep myself hydrated as I was breastfeeding and knew I needed to feed my daughter. However, I still always felt like I could have done a better job. Obviously, I know that going into parenthood is no walk in the park for anyone, although it can feel quite alarming for those who have ADHD and/or other mental conditions. How can you expect to prepare for something you've never experienced?! Through this change, I became aware and realised that this was all normal and all my feelings were valid.

I started using CBT which allowed me to change my thought processing so that I could put in place some healthy habits. My partner and I decided to download an app which kept us on top of food timings for us and the baby as well as meal prepping for the week. Don't get me wrong, this wasn't a quick fix at all. Late nights and early wake-ups made this very difficult, but we powered through with making the necessary changes. As discussed in chapter 8, it may be useful to be open with your concerns and ask for help and support when needed. Sometimes we need extra support from others when going through these changes, and there is absolutely nothing wrong with that!

Going into parenthood was another breaking

point I experienced in my life which made me start journaling again and keeping a diary close to me so that I kept on top of things. Eventually, my perspective on parenthood changed and I started seeing it as part of a journey in my life. And that's the point here, learning and adapting to the changes are all a part of your journey.

Holly, 28

"I decided to leave my job and start up my own small business... just before leaving, I decided to write pros and cons about it. This helped me a lot in making this change because I felt prepared knowing what I was getting myself into. It was very hard at the start, but I was a lot happier with this change in my life. Writing all my concerns down and having the support from my girlfriend encouraged me to make this change happen."

Changes are a part of life, but it is how we deal with them that makes us who we want to be. It is important not to see them as a threat, but to take them on as we always do with everything else!

Hormonal changes

Our hormones and period cycles can play a huge

part in how we perceive life and the changes we experience. Unfortunately, we can't control our hormones, but we can have a better understanding of them. In turn, we will be able to isolate how it impacts our traits and allow us to shift our actions to accommodate them. Having a period cycle whilst managing our ADHD traits can be frustrating at times, so just allowing ourselves a bit of breathing room when it comes to our forgetfulness or impatience can take a weight off of our shoulders. Don't be so hard on yourself.

Many women with ADHD, or traits of it, experience higher levels of distractibility and are unfocused on tasks during their cycles. With this, a shift in mood, as well as physical symptoms can feel all too overwhelming. During this time, it can make us question our ability to manage these symptoms and our ADHD traits at the same time. We are all human. This is something that should be normalised on our journey.

Women who are going through perimenopause for however long can feel like their symptoms are never-ending. Even many women who don't have ADHD have said they feel like they now have it. My Step mum can definitely vouch for this. Either way, many struggle more with their traits of ADHD whilst also going through these hormonal changes. This incontrollable change can make it more challenging for women to work in their usual working environments. A decrease in work performance for something that women can't control can leave them feeling discouraged and hopeless. Although more businesses are recognising perimenopause and menopause and are increasingly getting the information they need to help assist employees when going through these changes, some are still left in the dark or do not want to learn. That is why as a society, we need to speak up for all of us so that we can get the help and support we need to ease these changes.

Pregnancy is also another massive hormonal change that can affect our perception of life. Like many women do, I suffered from postnatal depression after the birth of my daughter. I felt like I couldn't manage anything anymore. My irritability and impatience increased. I was fortunate to have a good support system to help with my hormones. It was also recognised that I was deficient in iron which accounted for my irritability. When I eventually stopped breastfeeding 18 months later, my hormones changed again. However, this time I was more prepared, and I was more aware of the changes my body made.

Hormones are a b*tch. But like ADHD, it doesn't define us. We work with it to discover ourselves the best we can. Adding a 'mood record/tracker' and what you eat, when you sleep, and what you do in your journal, can give you an insight into the areas you feel most incapable. We can then analyse why are we feeling this way. Similarly, to a thought process method mentioned previously, why exactly am I feeling this way? Is it that time of the month, have I eaten well today, am I sleep deprived, or am I lacking the nutrients needed for my body to function? It is a <u>must</u> to constantly check in on yourself. Always check-in. If all these are accounted for and you still don't feel your better self, then seek the professional help you need for a better way to manage your symptoms. Whether that's exploring medication or talking to someone. Help is always there.

I feel as a society, we need to talk about these more, as well as mental health, even ADHD for that matter. No matter what obstacle comes into your life, you can face them and adapt to any changes that may arise. Be your own advocate and look after yourself. Get the support you need to carry on with the journey you are living.

Final word

I hope this book has shed some light on the person you are and how best your mind functions. Learning about yourself is the key to living a happy life. Once you figure out your chosen strategies, you will feel comfortable and confident with managing your traits. No two paths are the same. No matter what route you decide to take for yourself, whether that's non-medicated, medicated, or using both as a method. You are still taking the same direction by helping yourself.

The takeaway from this is to make the wanted changes step by step. There is no rush to get to your destination. You will get to where you need to be in time and with patience. Find the fun in your journey. I recommend writing down your messiest traits first. Then decide on your next steps. Write down all the things you want to change in your life and focus on the challenging obstacles first. What strategy do you want to try? The next steps come down to you.

From now on, if you ever catch yourself thinking negatively stop at the moment and question it. Why are you thinking this way? What can you do to change this? Alter it into thinking positively. Get yourself in that positive thinking mindset and continue to walk down that pathway. Have you created your positive thinking pathway yet? Remember, you choose what goes and what stays in your life. You have the power to get rid of bad habits and replace them with good ones. Adapt to what life you have, or the one you want.

This book started as an idea, and it's taken me over a year to complete! It was very overwhelming at the start. I had so much self-doubt. I was in the mindset that I wouldn't be able to take on such a big task with my other priorities. I didn't think I would stick to it, but I changed this into positive thinking. I completed a book because of the strategies I used. I just took it on as a step-by-step process and didn't put too much pressure on myself.

I knew I would get there in the end, but I needed to enjoy the journey I was on by dividing my attention between my priorities. I would set myself a daily task of giving my attention to the book for at least an hour a day. As this became a habit, I started increasing my time. Then on the days I felt motivationally challenged, I broke the week up and gave more of my energy to myself. I gave myself a balanced life so that I could enjoy the journey I was on. And nothing is stopping you either.

Nicole Skimming

I leave you with this quote:

> *"Your beliefs become your thoughts,*
> *Your thoughts become your words,*
> *Your words become your actions,*
> *Your actions become habits,*
> *Your habits become your values,*
> *Your values become your destiny."*

-Gandhi

Acknowledgements

There are so many amazing people I need to thank for making this book a reality.

My deepest gratitude goes to everyone who has shared their real-life experiences with me, and now with others, to encourage and reassure the life challenges people face every day. Without your courage and bravery, this book wouldn't have been possible. Thank you for removing the taboo of ADHD and having the voice to rewrite its definition.

Secondly, I smile as I write my thanks to my partner in crime, my dear Benjamin. Words will never be enough for the support you have given me and our little family. Thanks for being a shoulder to cry on when the road got tough. You have a way to take my stress away… most of the time. An extra thanks for being my proof-reader.

To my loving sister, Danielle. Not only have you been one of my biggest supporters, but you have also been one of my biggest inspirations. The struggle we had growing up together not knowing that we had ADHD, is a bond that we will always share. Thank you for always making me feel heard and understood. I hope I will always make you proud. I am so honoured to call you my sister.

A special thanks to my friends - Mel, Fanny, Saffy, and Eleni. Your kind, uplifting energy has motivated me to pursue this book. You have never excluded me due to any of my traits, better yet, we have shared many impulsive memories that I will always cherish. You have also kept me grounded when I was perhaps a little too overwhelmed. I will forever be grateful for your kind spirits.

A huge thanks to the person I look up to the most in my life, Kyla – my Step-Mum. You have always made me feel that I could accomplish anything if I set my mind to it. You have always seen the best in me which gave me the confidence I severely lacked in my teens. Thank you for being the ears to my troubles, ideas, and achievements. You continue to amaze me with your drive to tackle the day, it never goes unnoticed. You are my biggest role model and I hope I make you proud.

Next, I would like to give thanks to my remaining family and friends. You have all had an impact on my life to shape the person I am today. Thanks to my passing grandparents; Grandad John - for your childhood memories as you taught me the value of sharing stories, Nan Susan – for your determination and belief that I had a good future ahead of me, and lastly, Nanny Ellen – for your kind and gentle touch – I will never forget how pure your heart was.

Finally, to my dearest daughter – Luna. You are my biggest motivator and I strive every day to become the mother you need me to be. I hope I make you proud. My only job is to help you find your voice in this world and let you know my arms will always be open. I owe everything to you.

References

ADDitude. (2016). *'Famous People with ADHD.'* [online] Available at: https://www.additudemag.com/slideshows/famous-people-with-adhd/.

Cherry, K. (2019). *'Why our brains are hardwired to focus on the negative.'* [online] Verywell Mind. Available at: https://www.verywellmind.com/negative-bias-4589618.

Goffman, E. (1963). *"Stigma; notes on the management of spoiled identity."* Englewood Cliffs, NJ: Prentice-Hall.

Healthline. (2019). *'ADHD Music: How Music May (Or May Not) Help You Focus'.* [online] Available at: https://www.healthline.com/health/adhd-music#white-noise.

Healthline. (2021). *'Imposter Syndrome: What It Is & How to Overcome It.'* [online] Available at: https://www.healthline.com/health/mental-health/imposter-syndrome#causes.

Healthline. (2021). *'16 Science-Based Benefits of Yoga.'* [online] Available at: https://www.healthline.com/nutrition/13-benefits-of-yoga#3.-

Yoga-improves-mental-health.

J Russell Ramsay and Rostain, A.L. (2015). *'The adult ADHD tool kit: using CBT to facilitate coping inside and out.'* New York: Routledge.

NHS (2021). Benefits of Exercise. [online] NHS. Available at: https://www.nhs.uk/live-well/exercise/exercise-health-benefits/.

NHS (2022). *'Eating a balanced diet.'* [online] nhs.uk. Available at: https://www.nhs.uk/live-well/eat-well/how-to-eat-a-balanced-diet/eating-a-balanced-diet/.

NHS (2018). *'Overview - Attention deficit hyperactivity disorder (ADHD)'.* [online] NHS. Available at: https://www.nhs.uk/conditions/attention-deficit-hyperactivity-disorder-adhd/.

Ramtekkar, U.P., Reiersen, A.M., Todorov, A.A. and Todd, R.D. (2010). 'Sex and Age Differences in Attention-Deficit/Hyperactivity Disorder Symptoms and Diagnoses: Implications for DSM-V and ICD-11.' *Journal of the American Academy of Child & Adolescent Psychiatry*, 49(3), pp.217-228.

Safren, S.A., Sprich, S.E., Perlman, C.A. and Otto, M.W. (2017). *'Mastering your adult ADHD : a cognitive behavioural treatment program. Client workbook.'* New York: Oxford University Press.

Sickel, A, E., Seacat, J, D. and Nabors, N, A. (2014). "Mental health stigma update: A review of consequences." *Advances in Mental Health*, 12(3), pp.202-215.

Suni, E. (2020). *'What Happens When You Sleep: The Science of Sleep.'* [online] Sleep Foundation. Available at: https://www.sleepfoundation.org/how-sleep-works/what-happens-when-you-sleep.

Surman, C., Bilkey, T. and Weintraub, K. (2014). *'Fast minds : how to thrive if you have ADHD (or think you might).'* New York: Berkley Books.

Verywell Mind. (n.d.). *'9 Types of Toys That Are Good for ADHD.'* [online] Available at: https://www.verywellmind.com/types-of-toys-that-are-good-for-adhd-5272458 [Accessed 16 Sep. 2022].

Watson, S. (2012). *'Adult ADHD and Exercise.'* [online] WebMD. Available at: https://www.webmd.com/add-adhd/adult-adhd-and-exercise.

Wilens, T.E. and Spencer, T.J. (2010). 'Understanding Attention-Deficit/Hyperactivity Disorder from Childhood to Adulthood.' *Postgraduate Medicine*, 122(5), pp.97–109.

Women's Health. (2022). '*10 celebrities who live with ADHD on how the condition shows up for them.*' [online] Available at: https://www.womenshealthmag.com/uk/health/g38642452/celebrities-with-adhd/ [Accessed 5 Sep. 2022].

Young, S., Adamo, N., Ásgeirsdóttir, B.B., Branney, P., Beckett, M., Colley, W., Cubbin, S., Deeley, Q., Farrag, E., Gudjonsson, G., Hill, P., Hollingdale, J., Kilic, O., Lloyd, T., Mason, P., Paliokosta, E., Perecherla, S., Sedgwick, J., Skirrow, C. and Tierney, K. (2020). '*Females with ADHD: An expert consensus statement taking a lifespan approach providing guidance for the identification and treatment of attention-deficit/ hyperactivity disorder in girls and women.*' *BMC Psychiatry*, 20(1).

Printed in Great Britain
by Amazon